Larissa Jones

ISBN 0-9720682-0-1

Evergreen Aromatherapy
Salt Lake City, Utah

Aromatherapy for Body, Mind, and Spirit

Photography by Frank Lusk and Stewart Woodruff.
Layout and design by Frank Lusk.

"Ointment and perfume rejoice the heart"
—*Proverbs 27:9*

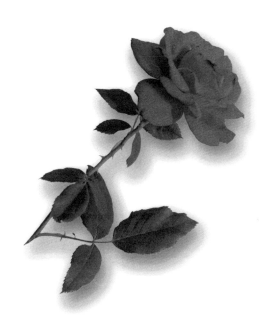

*The information contained in this book is in no way intended
to replace the advice of a qualified medical doctor.*

Much support and generosity of spirit has led to the creation of this book. I would like to thank the many Nature's Sunshine managers and friends with whom I have taught and laughed and who have supported me and my seminars. Together we have made a good thing happen. I hope aromatherapy brings balance and healing to you and your clients.

A special note of thanks goes to Ralph and Lahni De Amicis, Jim Crouch, Dick and Joy Williams, Richard Dicks, Bonnie Clayton, Angel and Jaqueline Giordano, Nanette Gil, Leo Batie, Linda Lee and Bobby Clark, Hannah Pavick, Jennifer Weiss, Carrol and Robert Knauff, Randy Anderson, Ruby Scherer, Dorothy Amstadt, Christine Takerian, Suzanne Bowen, Suzanne Wagner, Kathy Matschke and Anita Ramirez. Your friendship and support have made it all possible.

I would also like to thank Dale Lee, whose vision and program for professional education opened the door for the writing of this book; Beverly Lewis, who always speaks from the heart; Stacey Killpack, for frankness, honesty, and understanding; Kathryn Tuttle, for many times going the extra mile; Bob Shaffer, a friend and professional who tells it like it is; and to Gene and Kristine Hughes. I think the world of you all.

Thanks also to my fellow trainers for their support; to Greg Halliday and Craig Dalley; to Darlyn Anderson for her help, and especially to Frank Lusk for the hours spent working on this book's layout. And thanks to Steven Horne for forging the path.

My greatest thanks goes to my wonderful husband, Stewart. None of this would be possible without your love.

Table of Contents

8. Essential Oil Profiles

9. Aromatherapy and the Body Systems

10. Additional Materials

1

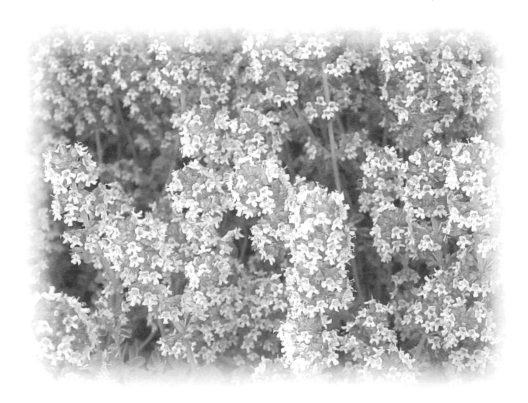

The History of Aromatherapy

The History of Aromatherapy

Pre-History and the Egyptians
The therapeutic use of aromatic plants may go back as far as 7000 B.C., when Neolithic peoples combined olive and sesame oils with fragrant plants to produce ointments. However, the Egyptians are generally credited as the true founders of aromatherapy. The extensive use of oils and fragrances required during the mummification process led the Egyptians to develop a vast knowledge of essential oils and aromatherapy. They prepared aromatic oils and unguents by placing aromatic plants in vegetable oil or animal fat and leaving them to infuse in the sun for weeks.

The Egyptians also practiced a primitive form of steam distillation using clay pots. They developed such aromatic extractions as cinnamon, cedarwood, frankincense, myrrh, juniper, and calamus. In fact, some of the work of these ancient Egyptian aromatherapists has lasted to this day in an unusual way. When King Tutankhamen's tomb was opened in 1922, a calcite pot in his burial chambers still gave off the fragrance of frankincense. More recently, as forensic scientists began to unwrap the inner bandages of a 3,000-year-old mummy, the aromas of myrrh and cedarwood wafted through the air.

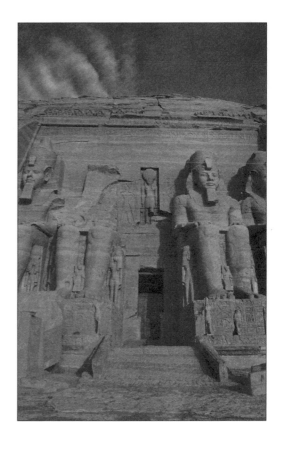

Natural aromatics were not only used during mummification to retard decay but were also burned as fumigants, used as medicines, and blended into perfumes and cosmetics. Legends tell of Cleopatra wooing Marc Antony with the scents of rose and orange blossoms. When she traveled to meet him, the sails on her royal barge were infused with the scent of rose, spreading the intoxicating aroma wherever she went.

The Greeks and the Romans

The use of fragrant oils has been documented in numerous excavations of Greek and Roman cities. The Greeks loved to use aromatic plants, and they laid fragrant materials such as mint leaves on the floors of their temples. Hippocrates himself recommended a daily aromatic bath and a scented massage in order to prolong life.

The Romans donned their heads with crowns, or "laurels," of fragrant bay (hence the term "bay laurel"), mint, and rosemary to commemorate important occasions and victories in battle. They were famous for their scented baths and fragrant massages. It is even believed that the name of the lavender plant came from the Latin *lavare*, which means "to bathe," because the Romans so frequently used lavender to scent their bath waters.

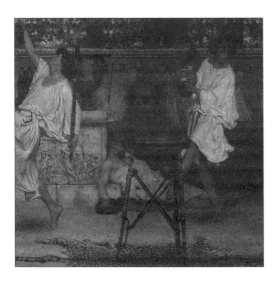

The Bible

The Bible contains more than 100 references to the use of essential oils. Two stories stand out among these. The first is the story of Mary Magdalene washing Jesus' feet, drying them with her hair, and then annointing his head with the expensive oil of spikenard.

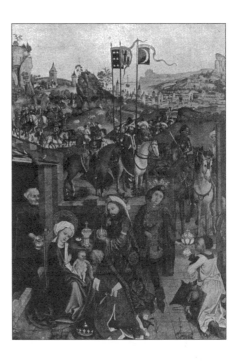

The second and perhaps most well known story is of the gift of the magi to the Christ child—gold, frankincense and myrrh. In ancient times, frankincense and myrrh were as valuable as gold. Because of the association of frankincense and myrrh with embalming and death, the gift of the magi is sometimes interpreted to represent life, death, and rebirth.

The Black Plague

During the 17th century, the Black Plague swept through Europe, killing more than one-third of the population. With the smells of decay, disease, and death lingering in the air, people sniffed pomander balls and carried nosegays to cover the odor. It was believed that the bad smells themselves carried the dread disease. Walking sticks with hollow tops were filled with aromatic substances, which were believed to ward off the plague.

Seventeenth-century French plague doctors covered themselves head-to-toe in leather and protected their faces with grotesque beaked masks. Inside the bird-like beak were aromatic herbs designed to protect the wearer from infection. It is from this strange costume that the term "quack" originated.

In London, perfumers and glovemakers who perfumed their gloves seemed to remain immune from the ravages of the plague. It is said that the city of Buklesbury, England, was spared from the plague because it was the center of the lavender trade. It is entirely possible that the antibacterial action of the essential oils that the perfumers and glovemakers were exposed to in their daily work protected them from infection.

The Birth of Aromatherapy

The term "aromatherapy" was first coined by French scientist Rene-Maurice Gattefosse. Gattefosse had been researching the cosmetic, antiseptic, and healing properties of essential oils when he severely burned his hand in a laboratory explosion. He doused the wound with undiluted lavender oil, which quickly eased the pain of his burns. His skin healed without any infection or sign of scarring.

During World War II, another Frenchman, Dr. Jean Valnet, advanced the science of aromatherapy. Valnet successfully used essential oils to treat the battle wounds of soldiers when drugs were in short supply. He later went on to successfully treat long-term psychiatric patients with essential oils and wean them off of their chemical medicines.

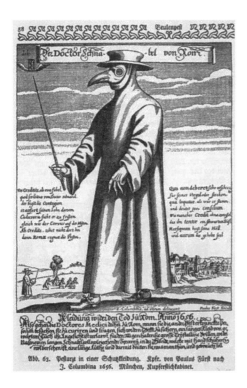

2

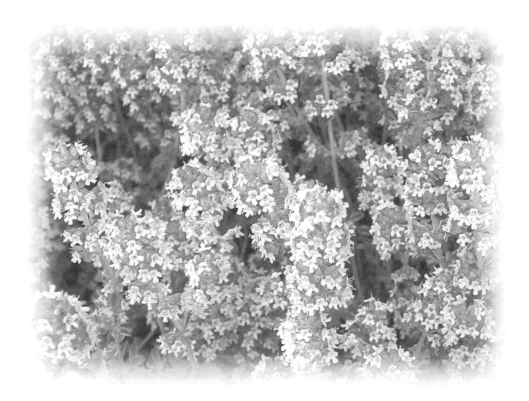

An Introduction to Aromatherapy and Essential Oils

Quick Definitions

A.O.C.—Appelation d'Origine Contrôlée, or Controlled Designation of Origin. This prestigious designation is given only to 100% pure *Lavendula angustifolia* essential oil grown in Provence, France.

Aromatherapy—The physiological and psychological responses of the body to the absorption (via the skin, digestion, or lungs) of essential oils and the use of pure essential oils for supporting the healing of the mind and body.

Biologique—The French term for certified organic, abbreviated as "BIO."

Carrier or Base Oil—A vegetable oil, skin lotion, or gel used to dilute pure essential oils before topical applications, such as massage.

Cold Expression—The process of obtaining essential oils from citrus fruit peels by pressure without the use of heat.

Dilution—The process of adding a small amount of essential oil to a greater quantity of vegetable oil, lotion, or other carrier to reduce the likelihood that a concentrated essential oil will cause skin rash or other irritation.

Distillation—The use of steam to extract essential oils from aromatic plant materials.

Emulsifier—A substance, such as soap, that allows oil to mix with water.

Essential Oil—A concentrated and medicinal aromatic substance derived from the distillation of aromatic plants. Essential oils are naturally found in specialized glands within the tissues of aromatic plants, and are used by the plant for immunity and chemical communication with other plants.

Nebulizing Diffuser—A mechanical pump apparatus that blows air through undiluted essential oils and disperses them throughout the air without the use of heat. A nebulizing diffuser disburses an invisible cloud of essential oil particles over an area of approximately 100 square feet.

Neat—The use of essential oils without diluting them in a carrier or base oil. The neat use of essential oils can lead to skin rashes and irritation. The only essential oil considered completely safe for neat applications is lavender. Although tea tree is also often used neat, a small percentage of individuals show skin sensitivity to neat tea tree.

Notes—Layers of smell within an essential oil, based on relative volatility. Top, middle, and base notes are explained in chapter six.

Volatile—From the Latin word *volare*, meaning "to fly." Easily evaporated.

Introduction to Aromatherapy

Aromatherapy is the use of essential oils to address various physical and emotional concerns. It is powerful not just because of its healing benefits for the body, but also because of its soothing effects on the emotions. Essential oils can work almost instantly, especially for hormonal and emotional concerns.

Smelling aromatic oils seems to activate the mysterious mind–body connection. The aromas bring us to a quieter state of mind so we can do a better job of taking care of ourselves. Essential oils awaken our natural healing intuition. Just by smelling an essential oil, our bodies will often give us feedback about how that oil will affect us physically and mentally.

Essential oils go to work immediately in the body because they don't have to go through the digestive system to get into the bloodstream. When you inhale an essential oil, the volatile molecules begin to be absorbed right into the mucosa of the sinuses. Other volatile molecules enter the lungs and are absorbed into the bloodstream through the alveoli, or air sacs. Thus, simply smelling or breathing an essential oil efficiently gets the essential oil into the bloodstream, where it can affect our physiology. Similarly, essential oils that

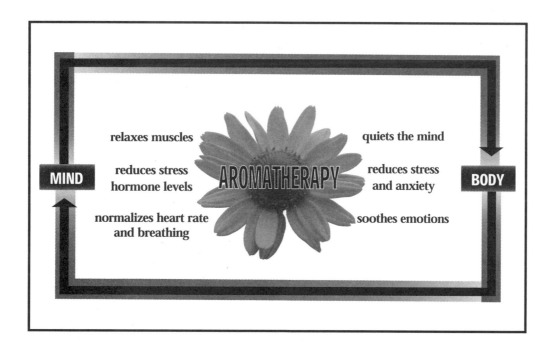

are massaged into the skin move through the skin and interstitial fluid and are absorbed into the bloodstream. Truly, the physical and mental effects of essential oils are harmonious and inseparable.

Definition of Essential Oils

Essential oils are concentrated extracts distilled from aromatic herbs, trees, and grasses. They can be located in various parts of a plant, including the seeds, bark, root, leaves, flowers, wood, and resins. Of the estimated 400,000 plants found on the earth, only a few are distilled to produce essential oils. Many plants produce only a minute amount of essential oil, and the sheer volume of plant material needed prohibits their commercial production.

Essential oils are volatile, meaning they vaporize quickly into the air. It is partially due to the vaporization of these molecules that we are able to detect the scent of aromatic plants. The term "essential" is derived from *quintessence*, defined as "an extract of a substance containing its principle in its most concentrated forms." Essential oils were named "essential" because they were considered to be the very essence, or spirit, of the plant. These oils are light and non-greasy to the touch. They are classified as oils only because they are soluble in fatty oils, such as olive or sesame, whereas they are relatively insoluble in water.

Pure essential oils are also concentrated, being at least 50 times more potent than the plants from which they are derived (Keville and Green, 29). The amount of essential oil contained in an aromatic plant is small compared to the overall weight of the plant. For example, it takes over 100 pounds of lavender to produce one pound of essential oil (Cooksley, 9). In some cases, using an herb may be safer than using a concentrated essential oil. For example, the herb sage is considered quite safe, while the essential oil of sage must be used with great caution, because it has a concentrated level of the neurotoxic chemical thujone.

> ESSENTIAL OILS ARE AT LEAST **50** TIMES MORE POTENT THAN THEIR HERBAL COUNTERPARTS.

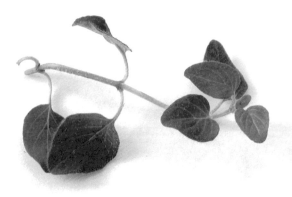

Olfactory Perception

The process of olfaction (the scientific term for smelling) begins when a molecule of odorant travels to the nose. The nose is a passage to the olfactory epithelium, a special mucous membrane located at the roof of the nasal cavity. Here, odors penetrate and dissolve into the mucus. Protruding into the epithelium are cilia—hair-like structures that are actually the tips of specialized olfactory nerves. These olfactory nerves relay information through the olfactory bulb deep into the "old" brain, or the limbic system. These olfactory nerves are considered to be part of the brain, so you could say that the brain extends outwards via the nose. Our sense of smell is the one place in the body where the nervous system is in direct contact with our external environment.

> OLFACTORY NERVES ARE CONSIDERED PART OF THE BRAIN, SO YOU COULD SAY THAT THE BRAIN EXTENDS OUTWARD VIA THE NOSE.

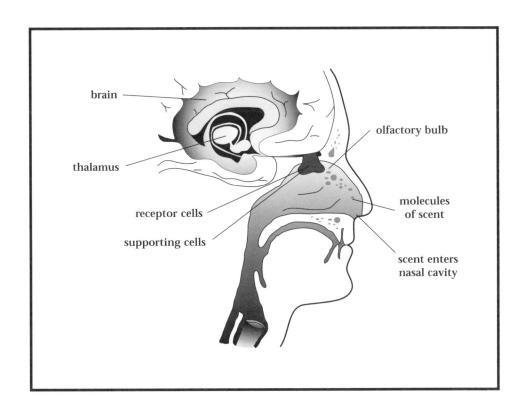

brain

thalamus

receptor cells

supporting cells

olfactory bulb

molecules of scent

scent enters nasal cavity

Emotions and the Limbic System

"Look in the perfumes of flowers and of nature for peace of mind and joy of life." —Wang Wei

Why do aromas touch our hearts and evoke our emotions? Why do fragrances bring back memories, and cause us to feel gladness, release, attraction and a host of other emotions? The answer lies deep in the brain in a structure known as the limbic system. The limbic system is considered by some scientists to be the oldest part of the brain, the part from which our cerebral cortex—the thinking, analytical part of the brain—is thought to have developed. Why is this distinction important? Because when the nose perceives a natural fragrance, this information is sent directly to the limbic system without having to be shuttled to other parts of the brain to be analyzed. Our reactions to the smell are largely involuntary, and our subconscious mind is more affected by aromas than our conscious mind.

The more primitive limbic system is connected with involuntary reactions that tell us about our perception of the environment via emotional and visceral responses. For example, if you open

and smell a bottle of milk that has gone bad, the rotten aroma registers instantly in the limbic system. Almost immediately your stomach churns and you physically move away from the milk. All of this happens without consciously telling yourself to become nauseated and move away from the smell. Your cortex just registers a highly negative reaction, and that response has an emotional basis within the limbic system.

When the limbic system recognizes pleasant smells, such as the smell of cookies baking, it instantly triggers a bodily response of relaxation and an emotional response of pleasure. This system is also responsible for recognizing chemicals known as pheromones, which affect mood and sexual attraction.

The hypothalamus is part of the limbic system. Its functions include synthesis of pituitary hormones and control of visceral and emotional responses. Together, the limbic system and the hypothalamus initiate primitive, emotional drives—sex and hunger for example—and evoke the visceral mechanisms causing gut reactions like rage, revulsion, fear, sorrow, affection and sexual attraction (Damian, 75).

Aromatic stimuli in the limbic system cause the release of neurotransmitters, including pain-reducing encephalin, pleasure-producing endorphins, relaxing serotonin, and stimulating noradrena-line. In describing the role of the limbic system, Susanne Fischer-Rizzi writes,

" Here is the seat of our sexuality, the impulse of attraction and aversion, our motivation and our moods."

It is possible to scientifically document changes in the brain caused by inhaling aromatic materials. We do this by meas-uring the electrical activity of the brain with an electroencephalograph (EEG). This machine records patterns of brain waves.

The aromas of basil, rosemary and pep-permint have been shown to increase production of beta waves in the brain, an indication of mental alertness and feel-ings of well-being. Test subjects exposed to these aromas were more accurate in their performance of set tasks (Walji, 18). The scent of lemon oil is also stim-ulating to the brain, and has been shown to improve mental concentration. According to Julie Lawless, a Japanese study demonstrated that typing errors were reduced by an amazing 54 percent when essential oil of lemon was dis-bursed in the room (Lawless, 18).

While some essential oil fragrances are stimulating and uplifting to the brain, others are relaxing and sedating. Pleasant smelling aromas such as clary sage and chamomile produce the brain waves associated with peaceful, relaxed states—alpha, theta and delta waves. Researches at the Toho University School of Medicine in Tokyo found that inhaling lavender and sandalwood will increase alpha wave activity in the brain. Researchers at the Tokyo University of Pharmacy and Life Sciences found that inhaling chamomile aroma reduced blood levels of stress hormones (Tucker, 47–48). The smell of spiced apple has been clinically proven to reduce stress and lower blood pressure (Walji, 18).

Holistic Healing with Herbs and Essential Oils

The practice of aromatherapy is a recent and powerful tool in the field of alternative medicine. However, using aromatherapy should be seen as part of a healing continuum and not as a stand-alone practice. While aromatherapy offers a great deal to alternative practitioners and clients, it is important to look at a person's treatment in a holistic manner.

Perhaps the best way to understand what role aromatherapy should play in your healing repertoire is to understand how herbs are processed. Distilling or otherwise extracting an essential oil from plant material is only one of many ways a plant can be prepared as a remedy. Herbs may also be made into teas and decoctions, tinctures or swallowed whole.

Extracting an essential oil from aromatic materials will concentrate some, but not all, of the healing properties of an herb.

Remember that essential oils are at least 50 times more potent than the original plant from which they were derived. These concentrated healing properties include antimicrobial, antispasmodic, anti-inflammatory, stimulating, relaxing and other actions that are more profound and immediate with the use of essential oils than with their herbal counterparts.

In contrast to an essential oil, herbs taken in their whole form have milder but more broad-ranging effects on the body, supplying not only essential oils, but also vitamins, minerals and other phytonutrients, which help to build the strength of the body as a whole. I think of essential oils as concentrated lasers, while whole herbs offer more comprehensive, but generally milder, healing properties.

For example, German chamomile is valued both as a whole herb and as an essential oil. A major constituent of the essential oil of chamomile is *chamazulene*, which imparts the herb's qualities of being relaxing, soothing to the skin, antispasmodic, wound healing and anti-inflammatory. Because of the concentration of the chamazulene in the essential oil, it is more suitable for topical use. In its whole form, chamomile only contains a small amount of chamazulene. Its other active components include tannins, bitters, mucilage and glycosides, all of which are pharmacologically active substances.

These additional components of the whole herb, along with its small quantity of volatile oil, make it a desirable choice for health concerns such as indigestion and colitis. The whole herb is also more appropriate for internal use. The essential oil, on the other hand, should be applied externally as a stomach or intestinal massage, where the stronger antispasmodic and anti-inflammatory actions of the essential oil are most beneficial.

Another example is sage. The common herb sage, *Salvia officinalis*, is considered to be safe for internal use. However, the essential oil of common sage has significant levels of a chemical family known as ketones, which are neurotoxic. Essential oil of sage must be used with great care and is not considered safe for internal use. Do not confuse the essential oil of common sage, *Salvia officinalis*, with the much safer essential oil of clary sage, or *Salvia sclarea*. Because of its relative safety compared to common sage, the use of clary sage essential oil is preferred in aromatherapy.

> THE HEALING PROPERTIES OF HERBS ARE CONCENTRATED IN THE ESSENTIAL OILS, SO THEIR ACTIONS ARE MORE IMMEDIATE. WHOLE HERBS PROVIDE MORE COMPREHENSIVE (BUT GENERALLY MILDER) HEALING BENEFITS.

Essential Oil Safety

Follow label instructions. Use externally; do not ingest.

Keep essential oils away from children.

Dilute essential oils before using topically. Undiluted oils may cause skin irritation. Essential oils do not dissolve in water and must be diluted with a vegetable oil.

Always keep a carrier oil readily available when using essential oils, in case of irritation.

Patch test essential oils on a small area of skin to determine skin sensitivity. Potentially irritating oils include but are not limited to eucalyptus, pine, cinnamon, clove, and lemon.

Generally, people with allergies must be very cautious with essential oils. The least sensitive area is the soles of the feet.

Essential oils, in their concentrated state, must never come in contact with mucous membranes, eyes, or sensitive skin areas. Milk can be used to flush the eye should contact occur.

Avoid exposure to the sun or tanning beds after topical application of essential oils. This is especially important with citrus oils.

Some oils have strong, caustic characteristics and should be used cautiously and in a diluted form.

Before using essential oils, consult a physician if you are pregnant, terminally ill, or undergoing drug therapy.

Periodically take a break from using essential oils. Use for six days and rest for one day, or use for three weeks and rest for one week.

3

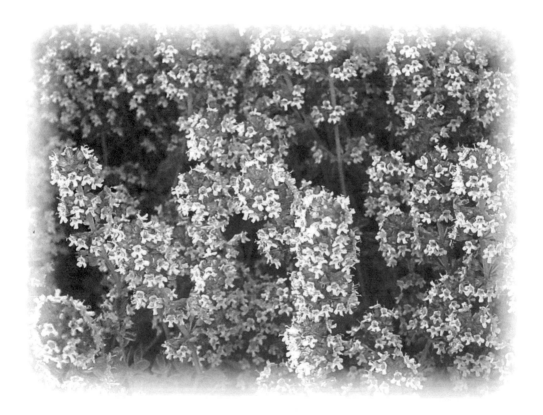

The Chemistry of Essential Oils

The Chemistry of Essential Oils—Quick Reference Chart

CHEMICAL FAMILY	ESSENTIAL OILS CONTAINING THIS FAMILY
TERPENES (monoterpenes) *Antiseptic, bactericidal, antiviral, drying, irritating to the skin.*	Lemon, Pink Grapefruit, Pine
SESQUITERPENES *Anti-inflammatory, soothing, sedative.*	Chamomile, Sandalwood, Vetiver, Patchouli
ALCOHOLS *Gentle, toning, stimulating, antiviral, anti-bacterial, energizing.*	Geranium, Tea Tree, Bergamot, Rose, Lavender, Thyme linalol, Peppermint
PHENOLS *Stimulating to nervous and immune systems, strongly bactericidal and antiviral. Potentially irritating to the liver. Irritating to the skin.*	Clove, Oregano
KETONES *Dissolve mucus and fats, assist in wound healing.* *Potentially neurotoxic and dangerous in large amounts.*	Sage, Thuja, Tansy, Rosemary
ESTERS *Balancing, soothing, antispasmodic.*	Ylang Ylang, Lavender, Roman Chamomile, Clary Sage, Geranium
ETHERS *Antispasmodic, digestive, licorice smell.*	Basil, Tarragon, Nutmeg
ALDEHYDES *Sedative, calming, lemon-like scent, antiseptic, antifungal, irritating to the skin.*	Citronella, Lemon verbena, Melissa, Bergamot
OXIDES *Expectorant.*	Eucalyptus, Rosemary, Tea Tree

The Chemistry of Essential Oils

Essential oils are complex mixtures of various types of organic molecules. An essential oil usually contains about 100 different types of volatile molecules. Some of these have been classified into larger functional groups that have predictable characteristics. The main groups are monoterpenes, sesquiterpenes, phenols, alcohols, ketones, esters, ethers, aldehydes, and oxides. Classifying essential oils into these chemical groups allows us to understand some of the basic properties and actions of individual oils.

Because any given essential oil may contain several of these different chemical groups, it can have a broad range of healing properties. Eucalyptus, for example, has stimulant, antiseptic, and decongestant properties because of its terpene, alcohol, and oxide content.

Monoterpenes (or hydrocarbons)— Because they form a chain made solely of carbon and hydrogen molecules, monoterpenes are classified as "aliphatic" rather than "aromatic." For aromatherapy purposes, monoterpenes are generally referred to simply as terpenes. Terpenes occur in virtually all essential oils and are generally mild.

They can be antiseptic, bactericidal, and stimulating but are milder than phenols. They can also be irritating to the skin, so they should generally be used with some type of carrier. Oils that are high in terpenes include lemon, pink grapefruit, and pine needle. Common terpenes include limonene and pinene.

CHEMICAL STRUCTURE OF LIMONENE

Sesquiterpenes—Perhaps the most difficult of the families to describe, sesquiterpenes can have a wide variety of properties but are generally antiinflammatory, soothing, and sedative. Sesquiterpenes are often found in essential oils distilled from roots and woods. Sandalwood, chamomile, and vetiver contain sesquiterpenes—santalol, far-nesol and bisabolol, and vetiverol, respectively. Spikenard is composed almost entirely of sesquiterpenes.

Alcohols—Monoterpenols are the most common form of alcohols,* which tend to be toning, stimulating, antiviral, anti-bacterial, anti-infectious, and enervat-ing. They are good, non-irritating ton-ics, and are an excellent choice for chil-dren and people with sensitive skin. This large category includes geranium, tea tree, bergamot, and lavender fine. The alcohol found in abundance in lavender is linalol; other common alco-hols are geraniol and citronellol.

The term "alcohol" in this case is the nomenclature of scientists and refers to a chemical structure, or molecular shape, in which one hydrogen and one oxygen atom have been added to a hydrocarbon skeleton. Scientific use of "alcohol" in essential oils should in no way be understood to mean drinking alcohol (ethyl alcohol) or rubbing alcohol (iso-propyl alcohol).

Phenols—These oils are highly stimulating to both the nervous and immune systems and are bactericidal, antiseptic, and antiviral. In large amounts or concentrations, phe-nols can be irritating and toxic, espe-cially to the liver. Oils that have a high

phenolic content include clove (eugenol), wild oregano (carvacrol), and certain chemotypes of thyme.

Ketones—Oils in this family are infre-quently used. They can be neurotoxic and can have serious side effects. When carefully diluted and used in modera-tion, however, they can calm, dissolve mucus and fats, promote wound heal-ing, and provide antifungal benefits. Tansy, wormwood, and sage are three essential oils high in the toxic ketone thujone. Nontoxic ketones are found in jasmine and fennel.

Esters—These oils are the most balanc-ing of all, are the safest to use, and tend to have a pleasant, fruity smell. They are commonly antispasmodic, antisep-tic, and anti-inflammatory. Many esters are also sedative and fungicidal. Their balancing nature makes them par-ticularly effective on the nervous system. Roman chamomile contains a number of esters not commonly found in other oils.

Clary sage and lavender also contain a high amount of the ester linalyl acetate.

Ethers—These essential oils are not very common but can easily be identified because they often smell like licorice. They tend to be antispasmodic, soothing, and sedative, and can aid in digestion. Basil contains methyl carvicol, tarragon contains methyl eugenol, anise contains trandanethole, and cedar contains cedryl methyl ether.

Aldehydes—These oils, which often smell like lemon, have a very strong aroma. Examples include lemongrass and melissa. Although lemon essential oil contains some aldehydes, it is classified as a terpene due to its greater concentration of terpenes. Because aldehydes can irritate, they should be diluted for use on the skin. Aldehydes are antiseptic, antifungal, anti-inflammatory, calming, and sedating. Bergamot is high in the aldehyde citral.

Oxides—This chemical family is noted for the presence of the molecule known as 1,8 cineol (eucalyptol). Because eucalyptol is mucolytic and may have antiviral properties, it is used for coughs and congestion. Oils containing 1,8 cineol include eucalyptus, rosemary, tea tree, and bay laurel.

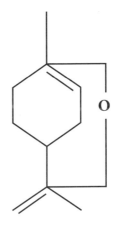

CHEMICAL STRUCTURE OF CINEOL

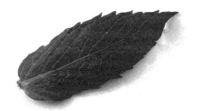

4

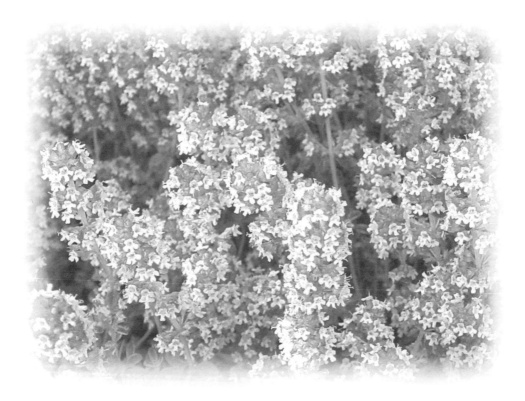

Ensuring Quality Essential Oils

Latin Names and Common Names

It is important to know the Latin name of the plants from which your essential oils are distilled. Latin names are based on a system of classification developed in the 1700s. This system is a hierarchy, starting with family, and then narrowing down to genus, species, subspecies, hybrids, cultivars, and varieties. The Latin name helps to avoid confusion, as many therapeutic plants have several common names, which may vary according to region and country. For example, the geranium used in essential oils has nothing to do with the red, potted variety that is also known as crane's bill. Geranium essential oil actually comes from the perlargonium plant, *Perlargonium graveolens*, commonly known as the rose geranium. Other varieties of geranium have odors of lemony citronella, mint, and chocolate.

Luckily, we usually only need to know the plant's genus and species, which are used to create a double name, such as *Lavendula angustifolia*.

Plant Species

In aromatherapy, it is especially important to be aware of the species of plant you are using. This is well illustrated in the case of lavender. Two types of lavender oil are widely used in aromatherapy: true lavender and lavendin.

True lavender oil comes only from the *Lavandula angustifolia* species. One of the most interesting experiences I had while studying aromatherapy was meeting with a third-generation lavender grower in France. This man explained with great pride how his family farmed lavender from seed, a traditional and time-consuming practice. He showed me how lavender grown from seed matures more slowly, but produces a richer, more complex essential oil than that grown from cuttings taken from a few plants. Lavender plants grown from seed take several years to harvest, and produce a soft, relaxing oil.

In contrast, lavendin, or *Lavendula hybrida* is a hybrid cross between true lavender and spike lavender. Lavendin grows quickly and gets much taller than true lavender, producing about twice as much oil. The essential oil from lavendin contains the stimulating chemical camphor, and although it is excellent for fighting colds, it has no place in remedies for relaxation, insomnia, and children's concerns. Both essential oils can be sold as lavender, and some manufacturers of lower-quality essential oil products blend the two types of oil to keep their costs down.

To insure that you are getting the highest quality lavender oil available, look for the correct Latin name and the designation "AOC" on the label. AOC stands for Appelation d'Origine Contrôlée, or controlled designation of origin. This certification was created by the French government and is given only to 100% pure *Lavendula angustifolia* essential oil, grown from seed in Haute Provence, France.

Location and Growing Conditions

While I was conducting research for this book, I had the chance to smell two samples of spearmint oil—one grown in Northern Morocco and one grown in Southern Morocco. The plants were identical except for the climates in which they were grown. But the oils smelled as if they came from two totally different species!

Every plant that produces essential oil has optimal growing conditions. For example, the best lavender oil comes from plants grown in the dry, limey soils and high altitude of Haute (high) Provence, France.

Every variation in the growing conditions of a plant—from soil makeup, to humidity, to temperature—affects the chemical makeup of the plant and changes the nature of its essential oil. When the chemical makeup of a plant and its essential oil are sufficiently changed by climatic conditions, the plant becomes a separate chemotype.

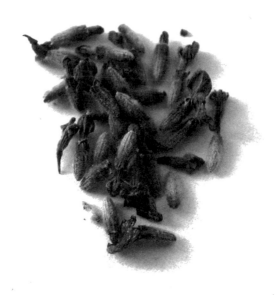

Chemotypes

When plants of the same species produce a different profile of aromatic molecules, they are called chemotypes. The difference in these chemical profiles is the result of weather, soil conditions, climate and genetics. Chemotypes occur naturally in the wild and are cultivated for their unique healing properties.

The species *Thymus vulgaris* produces eight different chemotypes. When thyme is grown at sea level, it is high in the phenol thymol and is designated as *Thymus vulgaris ct. thymol*, or simply *thyme thymol*. Phenols are irritating to the skin, and in large amounts they can be toxic to the liver. They possess powerful antibacterial proprties, but they must be used with caution and should not be used by children or the elderly.

When thyme is grown in the mountains, it is high in the gentle alcohol linalol. This plant is referred to as *Thymus vulgaris ct. linalol*, or simply *thyme linalol,* or sweet thyme.

Alcohols are generally non-toxic, non-irritating, stimulating and antimicrobial. In many cases, thyme linalol has comperable activity to thyme thymol, despite its lower phenolic content (Schnaubelt, 32). Due to the alcohol linalol, thyme linalol is much more gentle to the skin than the other chemotypes, and can be used by children and the elderly.

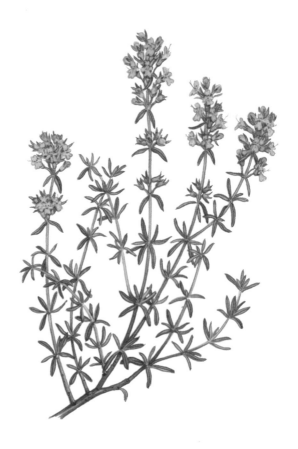

Gas Chromatography

One way to ensure the quality of an essential oil is through the use of gas chromatography, which separates the various therapeutic constituents of a given essential oil. A chromatograph is like a chemical "fingerprint," with the peaks showing the concentrations of the different healing constituents.

The chart on the next page shows gas chromatographs for two different brands of lavender. Brand A lavender is higher in two of the most desirable constituents, namely l-linalool and linalyl-acetate. Brand A lavender is more soothing and relaxing and has a softer smell. Brand B lavender is lower in the desired components and has a harsh, camphoraceous smell. In fact, Brand B lavender was "cut" with the less expensive hybrid lavandin. Since it takes about 100 pounds of fine lavender to produce one pound of essential oil, it is easy to see how unscrupulous suppliers might be tempted to thin down their essential oils with the cheaper lavandin. The same is true for Bulgarian rose oil, which requires approximately 4,000 pounds of handpicked flower petals to make one pound of essential oil (Cooksley, 9).

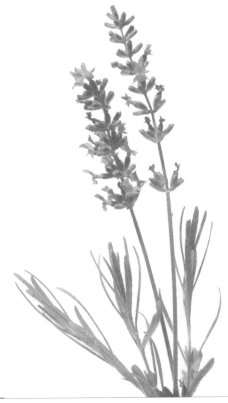

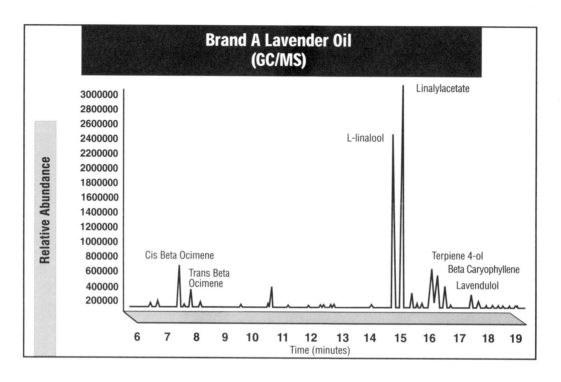

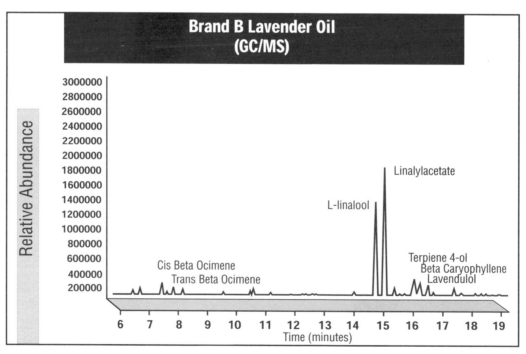

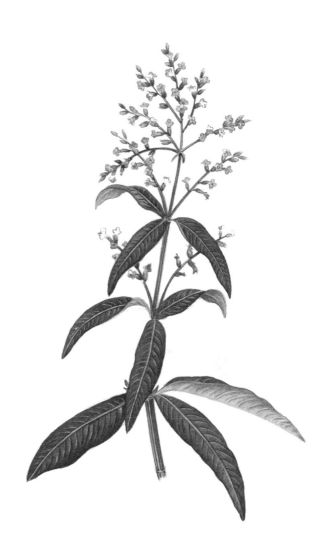

Learning How to Smell Quality

Aromas have distinct molecular structures that give them characteristic shapes. These shapes are perceived by our olfactory receptors, and the information is relayed to the brain. Two substances may smell very much the same, but have different molecular structures, and are thus processed differently. This is one of the reasons synthetic compounds do not have the same physical and psychological effects as their natural counterparts. In addition, people who have allergies and sensitivities to commercial fragrances often have no negative reactions when they use pure, high quality essential oils.

_5_

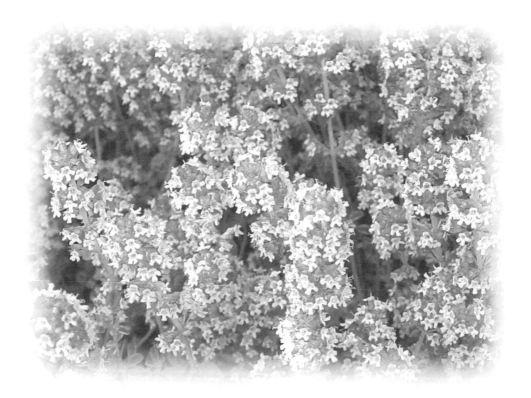

Clinical Application
How to Really Use Essential Oils

Ingestion, Inhalation, and Dermal Application of Essential Oils

Ingestion of Essential Oils

In a society in which we are accustomed to swallowing herbs and medicines, it is important to understand that essential oils are often most therapeutic when inhaled or used externally. If an essential oil is ingested, its therapeutic components will first pass through the liver before getting to the bloodstream, and some of its healing benefits will be lost. In addition, it is easier to overdose on essential oils by taking them internally. Although ingestion is sometimes the method of choice for trained aromatherapists, inhalations and dermal applications are preferable in most cases and for most people.

The chart on the opposite page illustrates the most appropriate methods of application for various health concerns. Notice that oral application is only mentioned for digestive concerns and immune concerns of the digestive system. Never take essential oils internally without the guidance of a trained aromatherapist and be sure to inform your doctor that you are using essential oils. Never take more than 1–2 drops of essential oils at a time and no more then 3–4 drops total in a day.

Always dilute essential oils in a carrier like olive oil or honey. Some essential oils are considered toxic and should never be taken internally.

As little as 10 drops of hyssop essential oil taken for two consecutive days has been know to cause seizure, and 30 ml of eucalyptus taken internally caused death in a 10 year old child (Tisserand, 52). I do not recommend the use of essential oils internally unless you are under the supervision of a trained physician.

Inhalation and Dermal Application

Essential oils enter the bloodstream immediately after inhalation and dermal application. When an essential oil is inhaled, the aromatic molecules travel into the lungs and then diffuse across air sacs known as alveoli into tiny capillaries. These capillaries branch out into larger blood vessels, and the essential oils quickly find their way along this route into general circulation. Inhaled essential oils have an almost immediate psychological effect because the sense of smell is so closely connected to the limbic system of the brain. Inhalation may be the best way to administer

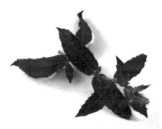

essential oils for the balancing of sex hormones, because of the aroma's effects on the limbic system and hypothalamus via the sense of smell.

When essential oils are rubbed onto the skin, the skin's own sebum facilitates their passage into the body. Essential oils then diffuse into the bloodstream or are taken up by the lymph and interstitial fluid. The rate at which essential oils can be detected in the bloodstream after a massage varies with the oils. Eucalyptus and thyme are two of the most quickly absorbed oils. Most carrier oils improve the dermal absorption

of essential oils into the body as does the friction of massage.

Essential oils are also excreted quickly from the body via exhalation, urine, feces, skin, and sweat. Again, the rate of excretion depends on the individual essential oil. According to Kathy Keville and Mindy Green, authors of *Aromatherapy, A Complete Guide to the Healing Art*, studies show that after a full-body massage with a 2 percent dilution of lavender in vegetable oil, detectable amounts of linalol and linalylacetate (the main chemical constituents of lavender) are found in the blood. Concentrations were highest after 20 minutes and diminished to undetectable levels within 90 minutes. "The study concluded that not only are essential oils lipophilic (fat-soluble) by nature, but that massage with a fatty oil accelerates absorption of essential oils by the skin."

Suggested Application Methods

Skin Care	Immune Concerns	Hormonal Balance	Emotional Concerns	Pain & Cramp Inflammation	Digestive Concerns
•Dermal •Baths	•Dermal •Inhalation •Oral* •Rectal/ Vaginal Baths	•Dermal •Spritz •Inhalation •Baths	•Dermal •Spritz •Inhalation •Baths	•Dermal •Baths	•Dermal •Inhalation •Oral*

*Under supervision of qualified aromatherapist; consult your physician

Getting Started

With the exception of lavender oil and sometimes tea tree, essential oils should not be placed directly on the skin. Because of their concentration, they must be diluted before application to the skin in order to avoid irritation. Essential oils are often diluted in vegetable oils, aloe vera gel, or lotion. The easy dilution chart on page 40 illustrates how to do this. The simplest method is to pour about 1/4 to 1/2 teaspoon of massage oil in the palm of your hand, add 2 drops of essential oil, and massage into the appropriate area, such as your neck or feet. As you get to know which essential oils are gentle and safe, you can use a greater quantity of them in the mixture, or you can use less massage oil.

One of the easiest ways to use essential oils is with a tea light warmer. This will usually be made of ceramic or stone, with a reservoir for water on the top and a place for the tea light below. Fill the reservoir with water, place several drops of essential oil on top of the water, and light the tea light. The warmth will diffuse the oils into the air. I look for units with large reservoirs so I don't need to continually refill them

as the water evaporates. Start experimenting with single essential oils and then with blends.

Use this soothing blend when you feel tired and drained.
>2 drops geranium
>1 drop frankincense
>4 drops bergamot

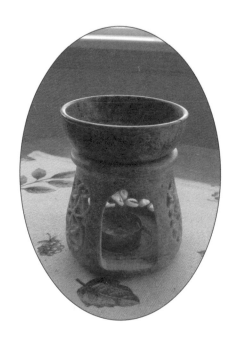

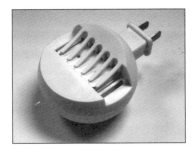

A plug-in wall diffuser gently warms and diffuses essential oils that you have dropped onto a rayon insert. It provides an easy and pleasant way to scent your home and remove odors from the air.

I also recommend that you pick up some spray or spritzer bottles. Glass bottles are best. Spritzers are an easy and effective way to use essential oils. One popular spritzer recipe helps calm excited or overactive children. I use this when my 7-year-old niece comes over to spend the night. Fill a 4 oz. bottle to below the shoulder with pure water. Add 6 drops of lavender, 2 drops of Roman chamomile, and 4 drops of bergamot. Shake before using. Spray on pillow and bedding, and spritz lightly in the air around your face and inhale. You can also use essential oils in spritzer bottles to make insect repellant, sunburn soother, and hormone- and mood-balancing blends.

Massages and baths are two of the most pleasant ways to get the healing benefits of essential oils. Suppositories and foot rubs are among the most efficient ways to get essential oils into the bloodstream quickly. Gargles and mouthwashes are great for colds, bad breath, and weak or infected gums.

As you become more serious about using essential oils, I recommend that you purchase a nebulizing diffuser. This is the best method of application for fighting airborne colds and flu, and respiratory infections. Vaporizors and steam inhalations are also helpful.

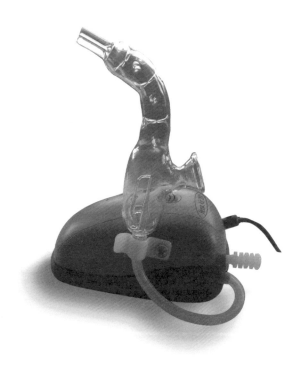

Application Methods—How to Use Essential Oils

NEAT

Essential oils that can generally be applied directly to the skin without diluting them first with a carrier oil include tea tree and lavender. Occasionally a person may show sensitivity to neat tea tree.

Acne

2 parts lavender
1 part tea tree
Apply directly to blemishes. For sensitive skin, dilute with aloe vera gel.

INHALATION

Essential oil blends can be inhaled gently yet directly from the bottle for a quick, emotional lift. For a deeper and more powerful inhalation, place 6–8 drops of your chosen essential oil or blend in a bowl of water that is almost boiling. Place a towel over your head and inhale for five minutes.

Nosebleed

3 drops lemon
1 drop lavender
Inhale from tissue.

DIFFUSION

Place 10–25 undiluted drops of essential oil or blend into the diffuser.

Pleasant Aromas

3 parts geranium
5 parts lemon
1 part frankincense
Combine the oils and add to diffuser.

VAPORIZER

Add about 10 drops of essential oil or blend to vaporizer water.

Cold and Cough Relief

10 drops lavender
2 drops eucalyptus
3 drops sweet thyme
6 drops bergamot
Add to water in vaporizer.

SPRITZ

Add 10–15 drops of essential oil or oil blend to 6 oz. distilled water. Shake well before using.

Hot Flash Relief

6 oz. distilled water (put in bottle first)
4 drops clary sage
3 drops Roman chamomile
3 drops geranium
1 drop pine
2 drops peppermint
2 drops lemon

SUPPOSITORY
Start with a base of Golden Salve.

Yeast Relief
    2 drops geranium
    2 drops tea tree
    2 drops lavender
    1 drop Roman chamomile
    1 oz. Golden Salve

Blend in a sterile 2 oz. jar with a sterile mixing stick. Form into finger-sized boluses and freeze to harden. Save some of the salve to ease external itching.

GARGLE OR MOUTHWASH
Add 3 drops of essential oil such as bergamot to a teaspoon of vodka. Mix with 1/4 cup of water and gargle. Do not swallow. Use just 1–2 drops if using stronger essential oils.

MASSAGE
Mix approximately 21–25 drops of essential oil into 1 oz. base oil. Apply massage blend externally, massaging toward the heart or applying to reflex points. See easy dilution chart on page 37.

Blood Pressure
    1 drop lavender
    2 drops lemon
    1 drop ylang ylang
    2 drops neroli

Blend into 10 ml massage oil and store in roller bottle. Apply to wrists or other pulse points 3 times daily.

BATH
Draw your bath, then add 8–12 drops of essential oil or blend to bath. Agitate the water in a figure-eight motion in order to disperse the oils, or try any of the bath additives on the page 37. Soak for 15 minutes.

You can also try a sitz bath by adding 5 drops of essential oil to just enough water to cover your lower body. For oils like lemon and grapefruit that may irritate the skin, use smaller amounts. See pages 36-38 for a complete description of bathing with essential oils.

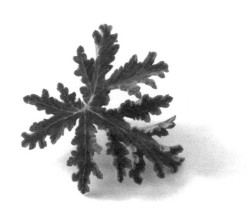

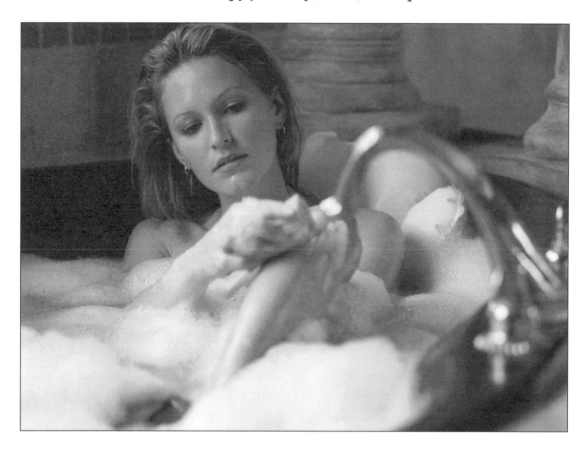

Aromatherapy and the Bath

Baths are one of the most pleasurable ways to use essential oils. You can use essential oils in baths to fight colds, revitalize your spirits, or help wash away the stresses of the day.

Baths with essential oils can be made even better by adding ingredients that will condition skin, soak out toxins, and ease muscle and joint pain. These ingredients also help disperse essential oils throughout the bath water. Dispersion is important because a large amount of an essential oil like geranium floating on the bath water can burn your skin.

For a lightly bubbly, cleansing bath, add 1 teaspoon of castile soap or Sunshine Concentrate. For relaxation, detoxification, or the folk remedy for sore joints, mix oils with 1/2 to 1 cup of Epsom salts or sea salt and add to your bath water.

ADDITIVES	AMOUNTS	BENEFITS	PRECAUTIONS
Castile soap	Quick bath: 2 teaspoons Bubble bath: 1/4 cup plus 1/4 cup glycerin	Cleans skin, prevents tub ring, disperses essential oils	Can be drying to the skin.
Massage oil	1/4 cup	Moisturizes lightly, disperses essential oils.	Agitate bath water. Be sure not to slip when entering and leaving the tub.
Jojoba oil	1/8 cup	Moisturizes deeply and heals.	Beware of slipping when entering and leaving the tub.
Epsom salts	1/3 to 2 cups	Detoxifies the body, eases muscle pain and joint aches, disperses essential oils	Do not use in cases of low blood pressure. Mix with essential oils before adding to water.
Sea salts	1/3 to 2 cups	Detoxifies, heals eczema, remineralizes the body, disperses essential oils.	Use caution in cases of high and low blood pressure. Mix with essential oils before adding to water.
Dead Sea salts	1/3 to 2 cups	Detoxifies, helps eczema, remineralizes the body, disperses essential oils.	Use caution in cases of high and low blood pressure. Mix with essential oils before adding to water.
Hydrated bentonite clay	1/2 to 2 cups	Detoxifying	May absorb smell of essential oils.
Kelp	1/8 cup	Detoxifies, contains minerals	Has a strong smell.
Honey	1/8 cup	Conditions skin, disperses essential oils.	Mix with essential oils before adding to water.
Milk	3 cups or more	Conditions skin, disperses essential oils.	Mix with essential oils before adding to water. Do not use if candida is present or suspected.
Apple Cider Vinegar	1/2 to 2 cups	Conditions skin, detoxifies.	None

Any of the bath additives in the chart on page 37 can be used with the recipes below.

Diuretic Bath
3 drops rosemary
3 drops geranium
2 drops lemon

Detoxifying Bath
4 drops lemon
3 drops thyme linalol
1 drop rose

Invigorating Bath
3 drops tea tree
3 drops pink grapefruit
1 drop peppermint

Refreshing Bath
3 drops bergamot
2 drops lemon
1 drop rosemary

Three Relaxing Evening Baths

3 drops lavender	3 drops sandalwood	3 drops lavender
2 drops rose or	1 drop chamomile or	3 drops geranium
3 drops bergamot	2 drops ylang ylang	

SITZ BATHS—Sitz baths entail using just a few inches of water—enough to treat the lower body. Sitz baths are used for hemorrhoids, painful periods, yeast infections in men and women, and other irritations or infections of the urogenital or rectal regions of the body.

PRECAUTIONS
The following single essential oils may irritate the skin, especially in hot bath water: ***clove, bergamot, pink grapefruit, peppermint, lemon, oregano, cinnamon and pine.***

Use no more than 1–2 drops of clove or peppermint and 2–5 drops of citrus oils per bath. Be sure to disperse these oils evenly throughout the bath water by using a carrier such as Sunshine Concentrate, honey, salts, milk, jojoba oil, or massage oil.

Massage

Touch has been shown to be important for mental health, immune system function, growth, and pain control. One of the best ways adults can enjoy the healthful benefits of touch is through massage. Massage can decrease stress hormones and the need for pain medications, and it can improve vagal tone, sleep, brain secretions of seratonin, and pulmonary function in children with asthma.

Essential oils can help to clear toxins from the body, open the lungs and sinuses, fight infection, reduce stress, and improve mood. Combine these benefits with massage, and you enhance the healing power of both aromatherapy and massage.

When using essential oils to enhance massage, you must dilute them with a carrier or base massage oil to prevent skin irritation. A base oil will also improve the absorption of the essential oil. Common base oils include almond, apricot, and sesame.

Follow the easy dilution chart (page 40) to understand the ratio of essential oils to carrier oil. A 1 percent dilution will provide a massage with a light, gentle aroma, whereas a 2–3 percent dilution will be stronger. A massage with a 4 percent dilution is quite strong but is sometimes used when a client is fighting a cold or respiratory infection, or suffering from muscular tension and pain.

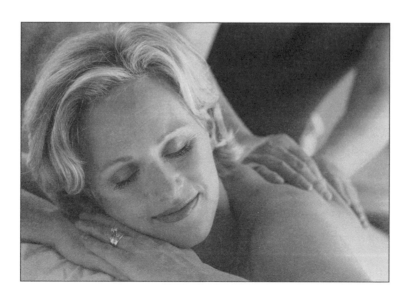

Easy Dilution Chart

SUGGESTED DILUTIONS FOR ESSENTIAL OIL MASSAGE BLENDS

Carrier Oil	Essential Oil		
Volume	1% dilution	2% dilution	4% dilution
1/2 oz. 1 tablespoon 15 ml	3 drops	6 drops	12 drops
1 oz. 2 tablespoons 30 ml	6 drops	12 drops	24 drops
2 oz. 4 tablespoons 60 ml	12 drops	24 drops	48 drops

DILUTION KEY

1% dilution is for children and the elderly.
2% dilution is for general, whole-body massage.
4% dilution is for concentrated, local massage.

The number of drops per ml of essential oil will vary based on the thickness or viscosity of the essential oil. One ml equals between 20 to 30 drops, depending on the reference used and the essential oil in question. I have chosen the standard of 1 ml=20 drops.

Remember that 5 ml is approximately equal to 1 teaspoon, which is approximately equal to 100 drops.

Reflexology

Another powerful method of applying essential oils is on the reflexology points of the feet. This involves massaging the energy pathways (or meridians) that move through the feet, thereby helping to move chi (or life energy) in specific body organs and clear energy blockages in the body.

Using essential oils either during or after a reflexology treatment may accelerate the healing potential of reflexology because essential oils also help to move blocked chi. Essential oils can be applied either neat or in diluted form to the soles of the feet in the areas that correspond to particular physical ailments. Refer to the reflexology map of the feet on page 42.

IT IS BELIEVED THAT REFLEXOLOGY ORIGINATED IN CHINA ABOUT 5,000 YEARS AGO. THIS DRAWING, TAKEN FROM AN EGYPTIAN PICTOGRAPH DATING 2500–2330 B.C., SHOWS A REFLEXOLOGY TREATMENT.

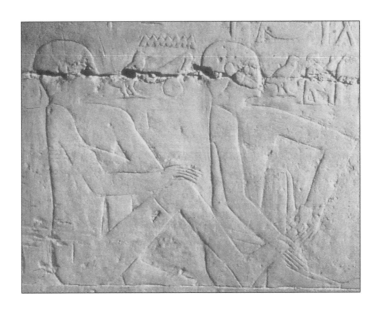

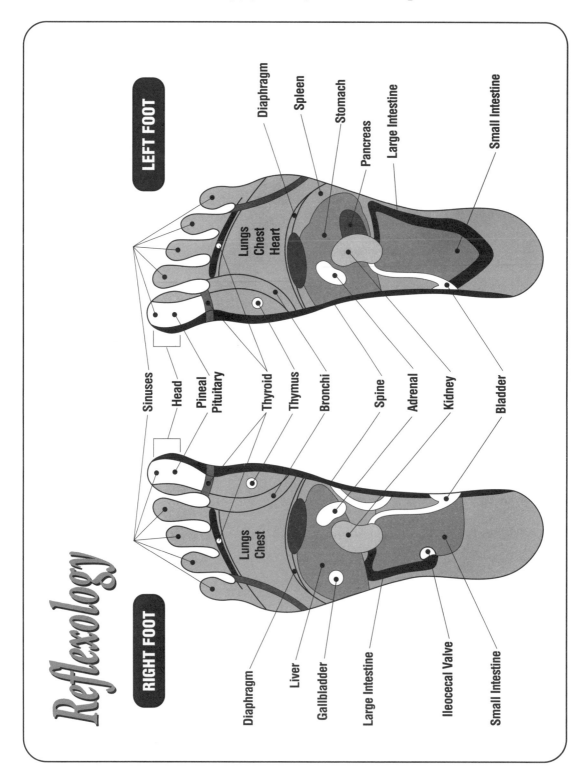

6

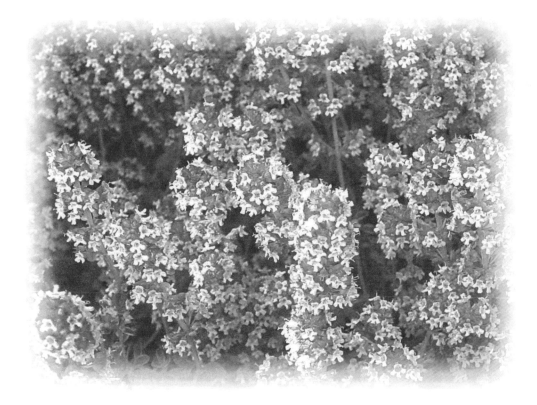

Aesthetic Applications
The Art of Blending

The Art of Blending for Fragrance

Every essential oil has its own fragrance characteristics. Learning how to recognize the smell of a good essential oil is analogous to learning how to taste a good wine. Essential oils have many layers of smell called "notes." The smell of a good essential oil can be described as organic and complex—unlike the flat, overly sweet perfume smells we are accustomed to in commercial cosmetics.

The art of blending essential oils is like creating a symphony. Combine the right fragrances, and you create a beautiful, healing, personal aroma that benefits mind and body. As you start to use and smell essential oils, you will begin to develop an intuitive understanding of which oils blend well together. Often you will find that you like the smell of a particular essential oil in a blend that you do not prefer as a single.

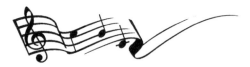

Although my personal preference is to make blends as pleasant smelling as possible, some blends developed specifically for aiding physical ailments may of necessity smell odd or medicinal.

Three Basic Guidelines

Blending two or more essential oils together can produce much more beautiful and pleasing fragrances than you

TOP NOTES	MIDDLE NOTES	BASE NOTES
Citrus Bergamot Grapefruit Lemon Mandarin	**Green** Pine Rosemary Sweet Thyme Clary Sage Marjoram	**Resin/Wood** Frankincense Myrrh Sandalwood
Green Tea Tree Peppermint* Eucalyptus*	**Floral** Rose** Geranium Chamomile Lavender Neroli**	**Floral** Ylang Ylang** Jasmine**
Spice Tea Tree Peppermint* Eucalyptus*	**Spice** Clove Cinnamon**	**Earth** Patchouli

* Top to Middle   *** Middle to Base or Base to Middle*

will find with any single essential oil. However, learning to make a pleasing blend is more of an art than a science.

To create your own, unique fragrance blends, consider these three points:
1. *The ratio of top, middle and base notes*
2. *The fragrance family and characteristics*
3. *The aroma intensity*

To begin to understand the fragrance and character of essential oils, you must explore the categories of top, middle, and base notes. Top notes are the most pungent and volatile. They act quickly and disappear quickly, their first impression lasting no more than 30 minutes. Top notes usually stimulate and uplift.

Middle notes are more stable. Their scent unfolds anywhere from one minute to three hours after application. They soothe and balance the body, and they round out a blend with softer tones.

Base notes are the least volatile and may be used as fixatives in a blend, holding in the fragrance longer than a blend without a base note. Base notes, heavier and thicker than other oils, are generally relaxing. They are deep,

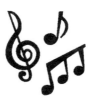

warm, sensuous, and often somewhat sweet-smelling.

One quick way to begin blending oils successfully is to use the following ratio: 3 drops of top note essential oil, 2 drops of middle note essential oil, and 1 drop of base note. Use this ratio as a rough guideline, and then adjust the blend according to your preference. Here are three examples of great-smelling blends that loosely follow the 3:2:1 guideline:

3 drops pink grapefruit
2 drops lavender
1 drop patchouli

or

4 drops lemon
2 drops geranium
1 drop frankincense

or

2 drops pink grapefruit
3 drops clary sage
2 drops ylang ylang
1 drop myrrh

> ### BLENDING GUIDELINES
> Top notes   3 drops
> Middle notes   2 drops
> Base notes   1 drop

Blending within Fragrance Families

Essential oils can also be categorized according to their fragrance family. Fragrance families often correspond to the location of the plant from which an essential oil is extracted. Aromas in the citrus family are pungent, sharp, sweet, and uplifting. Citrus aromas include grapefruit and lemon.

The aromas of the floral family are sweet, heavy, aphrodisiac, and, with the exception of jasmine, relaxing, sedative, and sometimes euphoric. Rose, ylang ylang, and neroli are all florals.

The herbaceous fragrance family is the largest and it is generally balancing and uplifting, with fresh, green aromas. Typical herbaceous notes are clary sage and peppermint. A subcategory of the herbaceous family is the camphoraceous family, which includes the more medicinal-smelling tea tree and eucalyptus.

The wood and resin families are always base notes and tend to be earthy, woody, or smoky in their aromas.

The final category of fragrance families is the spices. Spice aromas are pungent, warm, and lasting. Examples include clove bud, cinnamon, nutmeg, and cardamom.

I enjoy blending essential oils within their fragrance families. For example, the citrus aromas of bergamot and grapefruit smell great together, as do the herbaceous/floral aromas of lavender and geranium.

Aroma Intensity

Every essential oil has a different degree of pungency or intensity. For instance, patchouli is much more pervasive than many other oils. Just one drop of patchouli in a blend will make itself known, while a drop of lemon can easily be lost in a combination of oils. For this reason, it is wise to use relatively smaller amounts of high intensity aromas in our blends and comparatively higher amounts of lower intensity oils. This is not an absolute rule but a useful guideline.

If you don't want to take the time to learn how to make fragrant blends on

E
A
S
Y

B
L
E
N
D
I
N
G

C
H
A
R
T

Oil	Note/Layer	Blends with	Intensity (low use more, high use less)
Citrus Family			
Bergamot	top	neroli, lavender, geranium, chamomile, clary sage, jasmine	low
Grapefruit	top to middle	neroli, lavender, geranium, rosemary, clove	low
Lemon	top	lavender, ylang ylang, geranium, eucalyptus, sandalwood, rose	low
Mandarin	top	cinnamon, clove, lavend	low
Floral Family			
Chamomile	middle	bergamot, clary, geranium, lavender, rose, sandalwood	high
Helichrysum	middle	citrus, rose, lavender	high
Jasmine	base to middle	rose, sandalwood, clary sage	high
Neroli	middle	all citrus, rose, jasmine	medium-high
Rose	middle to base	all floral, clary sage, geranium, bergamot, clove, lavender	very high
Ylang ylang	base to middle	sandalwood, neroli, jasmine, orange	high
Herbaceous Family			
Clary Sage	middle	lavender, pine, geranium, all citrus	medium-high
Geranium	middle	lavender, patchouli, citrus, sandalwood, clove	medium-high
Lavender	middle	virtually everything	medium
Marjoram	middle	bergamot, lavender, thyme, peppermint	medium
Pine	middle to top	rosemary, tea tree, lavender	medium-high
Thyme	top to middle (linalol)	lavender, bergamot, marjoram	medium (linalol)
Camphoraceous Family			
Eucalyptus	top	lemon, thyme, lavender	high
Peppermint	top	marjoram, lavender, rosemary, lemon	high
Rosemary	middle	peppermint, basil, juniper, pine, lemon, cedar, bergamot	medium-high
Tea Tree	top	pine, ylang ylang, clary sage	high
Spice Family			
Cinnamon	middle	all spices, mandarin, ylang ylang, frankincense	high
Clove	middle	all spices, rose, clary, ylang ylang	medium
Wood/Resin/Earth Family			
Frankincense	base	all citrus, pine, geranium, sandalwood, lavender	high
Myrrh	base	frankincense, rose, pine, mandarin, geranium	high
Patchouli	base	rose, geranium, citrus, lavender	high
Sandalwood	base	rose, bergamot, geranium, myrrh, lavender, clove	low-medium

your own, the chart on page 47 makes it easy to blend for fragrance. Start by using the combinations already suggested in the chart. For example, cinnamon and mandarin always smell good together, as do lavender and mint. To use the chart, simply choose an essential oil, and look to see which oils complement it best in a blend.

Blending Recipes

FORTIFYING

    4 drops lavender
    4 drops bergamot
    2 drops patchouli

This blend can be enjoyed in many ways. It can be inhaled from the bottle, mixed with bath salts, or blended with 15 ml carrier oil.

SENSUAL

    2 drops ylang ylang
    2 drops geranium
    2 drops sandalwood

The addition of 1 drop of patchouli makes this blend richer and more interesting. A drop of clove makes it warmer.

This blend is too thick for a diffuser. Inhale or mix with 1/2 cup Epsom salts

and use in bath, or add 10–15 ml carrier oil to make a massage blend. Refer to the guidelines on the "Suggested Dilutions" (page 40) if you have questions on the dilution percentage.

STRESS RELIEF

    3 drops lavender
    2 drops bergamot
    1 drop Roman chamomile

This blend is excellent for all applications. Diffuse or mix with bath salts for a good soak. To make massage oil, mix with 10 ml carrier oil for a concentrated blend or 15 ml carrier oil for a 2 percent blend.

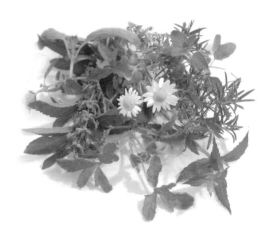

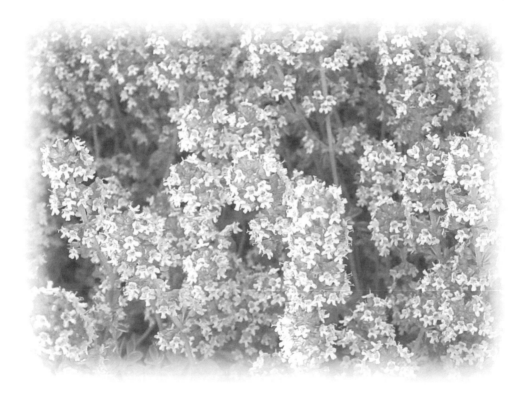

Aromatherapy and Emotions

Essential Oils and the Emotional Body

The effects of essential oils on our emotions can be powerful and numerous. To understand these effects, it is helpful to break them down into the following six categories: energizing, euphoric, stimulating, calming, grounding, and relaxing.

ENERGIZING: Lemon, grapefruit, thyme

EUPHORIC: Clary sage, rose, ylang ylang

STIMULATING: Rosemary, clove, oregano

CALMING: Lavender, bergamot, frankincense

GROUNDING: Patchouli, sandalwood, myrrh

RELAXING: Chamomile, sandalwood, lavender

These categories are not exclusive, meaning an essential oil can be both relaxing and grounding, for example. They are designed to provide a loose guideline to help you understand some overall characteristics of essential oils. However, the categories on either end of an arm of the star have opposite properties. Therefore, an oil that is calming is not generally stimulating.

Try smelling the individual essential oils associated with each category, and compare your body's reaction to each of these oils. See if you understand why patchouli is categorized as grounding, or sandalwood is categorized as relaxing, and so forth.

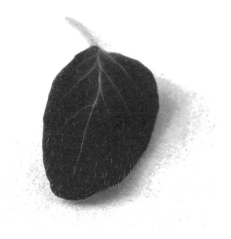

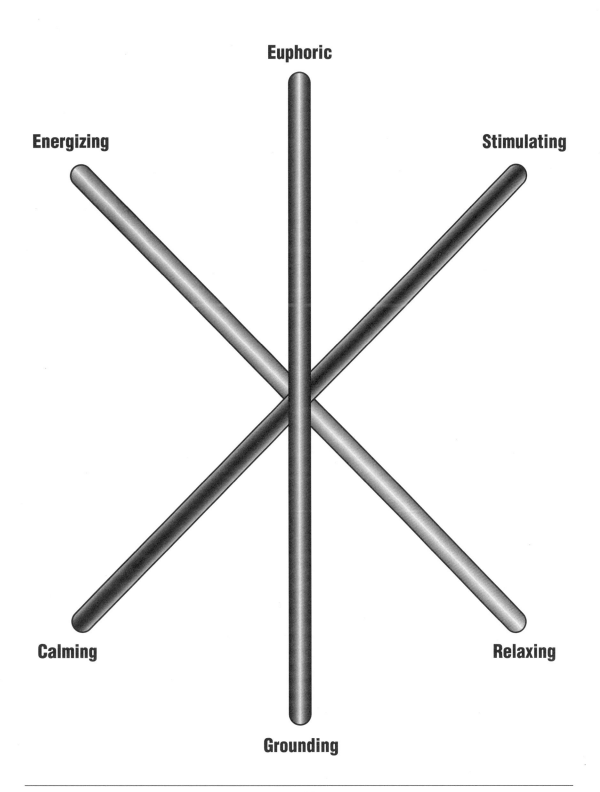

Aromatherapy and Emotions

A detailed list of which essential oils to use for specific emotional concerns follows.

ABSENTMINDEDNESS—Lemon, peppermint, rosemary

ANGER—Ylang ylang, clary sage, rose

ANOREXIA—Bergamot

AGGRESSION—Eucalyptus, lavender

ANXIETY—Clove, sandalwood, patchouli

APATHY—Pine, rosemary, tea tree, helichrysum

BETRAYAL—Peppermint, pine

BITTERNESS—Lemon, grapefruit, helichrysum

CRITICISM—Helichrysum, Roman chamomile

CLUTTER, EMOTIONAL—Myrrh, sandalwood, rose

CLUTTER, MENTAL—Pine, eucalyptus, clove, tea tree, lemon

COLDNESS, EMOTIONAL—Helichrysum, ylang ylang, rose, bergamot

COMPULSIVENESS—Bergamot, clary sage, patchouli

CONFIDENCE—Thyme, eucalyptus, pine, rose

COURAGE—Thyme, frankincense, rose

CYNICISM—Bergamot, sandalwood

DEPRESSION—Lemon, chamomile, bergamot, grapefruit, geranium

ENVY—Rose, ylang ylang

EMOTIONAL EXHAUSTION—Myrrh, pine, rosemary, geranium, chamomile

FEAR—Frankincense, rosemary, lemon

FAMILIAL PATTERNS—Eucalyptus, frankincense

GRIEF—Rose, bergamot

GUILT—Rose, sandalwood, ylang ylang

INATTENTION—Peppermint, tea tree

INDECISION—Lavender, lemon, patchouli, grapefruit

NIGHTMARES—Thyme, frankincense, lavender

OVERSENSITIVITY—Chamomile, pine

PARANOIA—Grapefruit, sandalwood

PROCRASTINATION—Grapefruit, sandalwood, patchouli

RESENTMENT—Rose, clary sage, lemon

SHOCK—Peppermint, rose

WEAK WILL—Pine

WITHDRAWN—Bergamot, ylang ylang, geranium

WORRY—Chamomile, lavender, frankincense

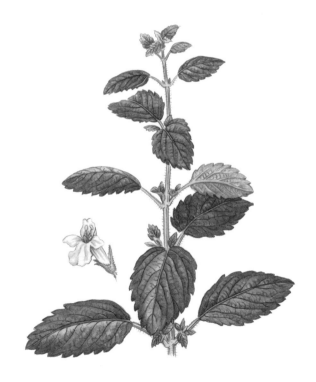

8

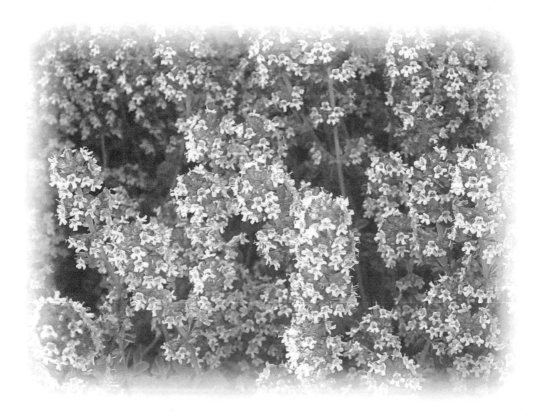

Essential Oil Profiles

Bergamot

Botanical Name: *Citrus bergamia*

Note: Top   **Odor Intensity:** Low

KEY USES:
- Addiction
- **Anxiety**
- Appetite loss
- Bladder infection
- **Depression**
- **Dyspepsia, painful digestion, colic**
- Eczema and psoriasis
- Gastroenteritis
- Insomnia
- **Intestinal infection/parasites**
- Mouth infection, herpes

Aroma: A blend of sweet floral with citrus top note and an undertone of vanilla.

Blends well with: Most other oils, especially frankincense, geranium, lavender, clary sage and cypress.

Part used: Peel

Properties: Antibacterial, antidepressant, antiseptic, anti-infectious, antispasmodic, anti-toxic, deodorant, febrifuge, stomachic, vermifuge.

Emotional concerns: Bergamot is helpful in cases of addiction, anorexia, bulimia, depression, fear, anxiety, and stress.

Contraindications: Bergamot is extremely photosensitizing and possibly irritating to sensitive skin. Do not expose skin to sunlight or tanning beds for 12 hours after use.

The bergamot fruit, developed for its scent, has been used in perfumery and medicine in France since the 16th century. Bergamot essence is mentioned in many old manuscripts and herbals. Bergamot is the flavoring used to make Earl Grey tea. The citrus bergamot should not be confused with bergamot herb, a red perennial also known as Oswego tea.

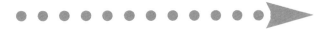

Bergamot is primarily used in aromatherapy for its antiseptic properties, which are in some cases as effective as lavender. Bergamot has a wonderful smell and can be used to improve the odor of antiseptic blends in a diffuser.

Bergamot is perhaps one of the most useful oils for helping with emotional balance. Its gentle smell is uplifting and opening without being too aggressive.

ANXIETY BLEND

8 drops bergamot
3 drops clary sage
2 drops geranium
5 drops frankincense

Mix oils in an amber glass bottle. Diffuse after a stressful day.

MOUTH ULCERS

4 drops bergamot
2 drops peppermint or 1 drop myrrh
2 drops geranium
2 drops thyme

Dilute in 2 teaspoons brandy. To use, add 1 teaspoon of mixture to warm water and swish well around mouth. *Do not swallow.*

Chamomile, Roman   **Botanical Name:** *Chamaemelum nobile*

Note: Middle   **Odor Intensity:** Extremely High

KEY USES:
- Anemia
- Anger and agitation
- Arthritis, bursitis
- **Cramps**, intestinal and menstrual
- **Children's ailments**
- **Dyspepsia, indigestion, flatulence**
- Eczema and psoriasis
- Gout
- **Insomnia**
- Irritability
- Liver congestion
- **Migraine**
- **Muscular aches, pains, tension**
- Nervous excitability
- Neuralgia
- Scanty periods
- **Sciatica**
- **Sedative (especially for children)**
- **Spastic colon**
- Teething
- Renal inflammation

Aroma: Warm, round, earthy, sweet, with a hint of green apple.

Blends well with: Sandalwood, rose, lavender, neroli, geranium.

Part used: Flowers

Properties: Analgesic, anti-anemic, antispasmodic, anti-inflammatory, calmative, emmenagogue, hepatic, sedative, stomachic, vulnerary, vermifuge.

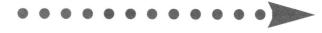

Emotional concerns: Chamomile is good for all states of agitation and anger, including nervous irritability, impatience, and oversensitivity. Chamomile dispels tension and fear. It is useful for people who tend to think, worry, or work too much.

The Roman chamomile herb has been used in European medicine for more than 2,000 years. In herbal medicine, chamomile is used for nervous tension, upset stomach, and children's ailments.

Roman chamomile essential oil is one of the best calming, anti-inflammatory, and anti-spasmodic essential oils. It is a good disinfectant for the urinary tract, and it soothes renal inflammation. Chamomile is also good for any skin irritation—rashes, acne, dermatitis, eczema, psoriasis, and itching. It is excellent for soothing burns and reducing scarring, and for soothing sore nipples.

TEETHING RELIEF
1 tablespoon olive oil
1 drop Roman chamomile

Mix essential oil and olive oil in an amber glass bottle with a dropper. Rub a small amount into affected gums.

NECK AND SHOULDER RELIEF
6 drops Roman chamomile
18 drops lavender
15 ml carrier oil

Combine in glass bottle. Massage into tense muscles.

Cinnamon

Botanical Name: *Cinnamomum zeylancium*

Note: Middle   **Odor Intensity:** High

KEY USES: (LEAF AND BARK OIL)

- **Candida**
- **Colds and flu**
- Digestion, sluggish
- Indigestion, Dyspepsia
- Infection
- **Infectious diseases**
- Muscle pain
- Nervous exhaustion
- **Parasites**

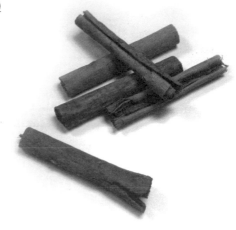

Leaf
- Lice, scabies
- Immunostimulant

Bark
- Childbirth
- Diabetes
- Severe infection

Aroma: Spicy, hot, sweet, sharp. Cinnamon leaf has a clove-like smell.

Blends well with: Mandarin, frankincense, ylang ylang.

Parts used: Bark or leaves

Properties: Anthelmintic, antidiarrheal, antimicrobial, antiputrescent, astringent, aphrodisiac, digestive, emmenagogue, hemostatic, parasiticide, spasmolytic, stimulant, stomachic, vermifuge.

Emotional concerns: Frigidity, faintness, depression, nervous exhaustion.

Contraindications: Cinnamon is a skin irritant. Use sparingly and never use undiluted. Do not use during pregnancy or on small children. The eugenol content in cinnamon may inhibit blood clotting. Do not use on people with slow blood clotting, hemophilia or those who are taking warfarin or other blood thinners. Do not use concurrently with Tylenol (acetominophen). Do not use in cases of liver or kidney disease (Tisserand, 66).

Cinnamon is one of the oldest spices known to man. It was a valuable commodity in the spice trade. The Egyptians used cinnamon as perfume, incense and medicine. The Arabs considered cinnamon a symbol of wealth, and it is said that Alexander the Great knew he was near the coast of Arabia when he could smell the spices from the shore wafting past his barge. Diffusing the essential oil of cinnamon leaf disperses unwanted smells and prevents the spread of infection.

The leaf and the bark of the cinnamon tree each yield essential oils that are chemically different. Cinnamon leaf oil contains a high percentage of the phenol eugenol, also found in clove. This may irritate the liver in repeated doses. It has a milder smell, and can be used in diluted form in topical and perfume applications. Cinnamon leaf oil makes pleasant aromatic diffuser blends and works well to combat sleepiness. Cinnamon bark oil contains cinnamic aldehyde, which is an excellent infection fighter. This makes cinnamon bark the oil of choice for severe infections. Cinnamon bark oil is also effective for stimulating menstruation and helping with uterine contractions during childbirth (Price, 79). However, the bark oil is quite irritating to the skin and should not be used topically.

Both essential oils are excellent antifungals, antivirals and antibacterials. They stimulate digestion and may be used to destroy intestinal parasites.

AROMATIC CINNAMON IMMUNITY BLEND
3 drops cinnamon leaf
2 drops frankincense
3 drops mandarin
1 drop myrrh

Place on cotton pad of wall diffuser. Or dilute in 1 ounce of massage oil for an aromatic, immune-stimulating massage.

MUSCLE PAIN RELIEVER
4 drops cinnamon
5 drops marjoram
3 drops roman chamomile

Mix with 2 ounces massage oil and rub into sore muscles.

Clary Sage

Botanical Name: *Salvia sclarea*

Note: Middle   **Odor Intensity:** Medium

KEY USES:
- **Anxiety**
- Asthma
- **Amenorrhea**
- Aphrodisiac
- Dysmenorrhea
- Dandruff
- Nervous tension
- **Hemorrhoids**
- Hypertension
- Intestinal cramps, colic
- **Menopause, hot flashes**
- Muscular tension, aches, strains
- PMS
- **Sweating, excessive**

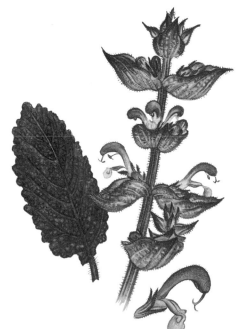

Aroma: Clean, nutty, sweet, warm, green.

Blends well with: Geranium, lavender, bergamot, sandalwood, rose.

Part used: Leaves and flowering tops

Properties: Anticonvulsive, antiseptic, antispasmodic, aphrodisiac, cicatrizant, emmenagogue, euphoric, hypotensive, sedative.

Emotional concerns: Clary sage is indicated for nervous anxiety, shallow breathing, depression and nervous tension. It is also helpful for emotional confusion and indecision. Clary sage, considered a euphoric, should be used only in moderate doses.

Contraindications: Do not use during pregnancy. Do not use while drinking alcoholic beverages, as this may increase the narcotic effect. Overuse can cause headache and stupor. Avoid using in cases of low blood pressure and estrogen-dependent tumors.

Clary sage was highly esteemed for its healing properties in the Middle Ages. Medieval authors referred to it as "clear eyes," because the mucilage from its seeds was used to clear the eyes of foreign particles.

Clary sage may be helpful in reducing high blood pressure, and because of its antispasmodic properties, it is helpful in treating asthma and muscle strain. Clary sage is also useful in addressing conditions of female hormone imbalance, including excessive sweating associated with menstruation or menopause, infrequent or scanty periods, and hot flashes.

Clary sage is also indicated for dandruff and hair loss. It can encourage vivid dreaming and improve dream recall.

HOT FLASH RELIEF
6 oz. distilled water
4 drops clary sage
3 drops Roman chamomile
3 drops geranium
2 drops lemon
1 drop pine
2 drops peppermint

Pour water into a spray bottle. Add essential oils. Shake to mix, and always shake before spraying. When you feel a hot flash coming, spritz yourself and inhale, or spritz a cloud of the mixture and walk through it.

PMS ABDOMEN RUB
3 drops lavender
2 drops Roman chamomile
2 drops geranium
3 drops clary sage
5 drops sandalwood

Mix with 30 ml carrier oil and massage into abdomen.

Clove Bud

Botanical Name: *Eugenia caryophllata*

Note: Middle   **Odor Intensity:** Medium

KEY USES:
- Amnesia, mental debility
- Colds, preventative
- Digestive disorders—dyspepsia, flatulence, diarrhea
- **Exhaustion**
- Expectorant
- Insect repellant
- **Mouth and tooth infections**
- Nausea
- Neuralgia
- **Parasites**
- Pulmonary infections (tuberculosis)
- Rheumatic pain
- **Sciatica**
- Shingles (internal use)
- **Sinusitis**
- Sore throat
- **Toothache**

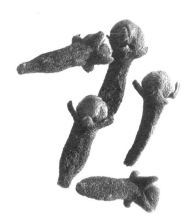

Aroma: Sweet, spicy, warm, penetrating.

Blends well with: Mandarin, geranium, sandalwood, cinnamon, lemon, rosemary,

Part used: Immature flower

Properties: Analgesic, antiparasitic, antiseptic, antineuralgic, antispasmodic, carminative, cicatrizing, stimulant, stomachic, vermifuge.

Emotional concerns: Clove is reputed to stop "mental chatter" and is good for emotional exhaustion, mental fatigue, and lack of concentration due to mental clutter.

Contraindications: The eugenol content in clove may inhibit blood clotting. Do not use on people with slow blood clotting, hemophilia or those who are taking warfarin or other blood thinners. Do not use concurrently with Tylenol (acetominophen). Do not use in cases of liver or kidney disease (Tisserand, 66).

Clove may irritate skin and cause contact dermatitis. It may also irritate the liver. It should not be used for long periods of time. Clove can be adulterated with other oils, such as oil of pimento. Be sure to use only high quality clove bud oil. Because irritation of the eyes may occur from airborne diffusion, do not use in the diffuser for more than a minute or two.

Clove is an evergreen tree native to the Moluccas in Indonesia. Their pink flower buds are picked just before opening and laid out to dry in the sun until they turn brown. Many old texts list clove as a stomachic, carminative, and digestive. It reduces flatulence, restores appetite, stimulates digestion, and fights intestinal parasites and viral infections. Hildegard of Bingen wrote that clove could be used for headaches, migraines, and dropsy.

Because of its high eugenol content, clove is an extremely powerful antiseptic—in some cases more powerful than oregano and thyme. Clove can be used in small amounts for short periods of time in inhalations or diffusions to fight colds. Be sure to keep your eyes closed or covered to prevent irritation.

BUG REPELLANT RUB
3 drops lavender
4 drops geranium
3 drops eucalyptus
2 drops lemon
1 drop peppermint
1 drop clove

Add to 1 oz. of carrier oil and apply liberally to skin. Eliminate the lemon if you will be out in the sun.

Eucalyptus

Botanical Name: *Eucalyptus globulus*

Note: Top   **Odor Intensity:** Very High

KEY USES:
- **Air purifier**
- **Antiseptic**
- Arthritis, rheumatoid and osteo
- Bronchitis
- Chicken pox
- Mind clearer
- **Colds and flu**
- **Coughs**
- **Decongestant**
- Diabetes
- Fevers
- Insect repellent
- Muscle aches, stiffness
- Neuralgia
- **Parasites, intestinal**
- **Respiratory infections**
- **Sinus infection, sinus congestion**
- Wounds and burns

Aroma: Camphoraceous, pungent, penetrating, fresh, with a slight woody/sweet undertone.

Blends well with: Thyme linalol, pine, lavender, lemon, marjoram, rosemary, tea tree, grapefruit.

Part used: Leaves

Properties: Antiseptic, analgesic, antibacterial, antifungal, anti-infectious, antiviral, bactericide, deodorant, decongestant, diuretic, expectorant, febrifuge.

Emotional concerns: Constricted, overwhelmed, feeling hemmed in and limited.

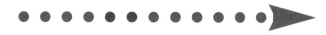

Contraindications: Eucalyptus may interfere with homeopathic remedies. Beware of rectified oil. Do not use in large concentrations on the skin. Avoid in cases of epilepsy or hypertension, and exercise caution in case of asthma.

Eucalyptus trees are native to Australia and are commonly known as gum trees. Since the late 1800s, eucalyptus oil has been used in remedies to treat coughs and other concerns of the respiratory system.

Eucalyptus is a powerful decongestant and expectorant and is therefore useful in inhalations in cases of colds, catarrh, and respiratory infections. It is specific for colds accompanied by chills and thin mucus. Eucalyptus is one of the best oils to use in a diffuser to prevent the airborne transmission of illness.

Massages with eucalyptus can reduce fevers and relieve the pain of muscle strain and rheumatism. Using eucalyptus on the dressing of a wound will speed healing.

ANTI-INFECTIOUS CHEST RUB
10 drops eucalyptus
4 drops peppermint
6 drops pine (wheezy cough, white mucus) or rosemary (catarrhal cough)

Combine in 1 oz. aloe vera gel, plus 1/8 teaspoon massage oil. Massage into chest and lower neck.

CLEANER AIR
6 drops eucalyptus
4 drops lemon
3 drops thyme linalol

Add to 6 oz. water in a glass spray bottle. Spray to freshen the air, or put oils directly into a nebulizing diffuser and diffuse.

Frankincense

Botanical Name: *Boswellia carteri*

Note: Base   **Odor Intensity:** High

KEY USES:

- **Aging skin, wrinkles**
- Asthma
- Bronchitis
- Calming
- Colds and coughs
- Cystic breasts
- Dermatitis
- Diarrhea
- **Emphysema**
- Fear, nightmares
- Painful periods
- Respiratory congestion, infections
- **Skin—scars, infections, boils**
- **Spiritual aid**
- Ulcers
- Varicose veins
- Wound healing

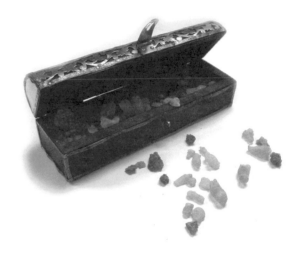

Aroma: Balsamic, woody, dry with notes of terpentine, rich, incense-like.

Blends well with: All citrus, especially bergamot and lemon, cinnamon, geranium, pine, rose, sandalwood, lavender.

Part used: Resin

Properties: Antiseptic, sedative, tonic, expectorant, cicatrizant, astringent, anti-inflammatory, relaxant, hemostatic, vulnerary.

Emotional concerns: Frankincense is opening, relaxing, and fear-relieving. It soothes the spirit as it deepens the breathing.

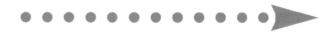

Contraindications: Avoid during pregnancy.

Frankincense, also known as olibanum, is an aromatic gum resin obtained from African and Middle Eastern trees. When the bark of the frankincense tree is damaged or deliberately cut, the tree exudes its resin, or "tears." The essential oil is steam-distilled from the gum resin.

Frankincense, one of the three gifts of the Magi to the infant Jesus, has been used since ancient times in religious rituals. Frankincense slows and deepens the breath, produces feelings of calm, and puts us in the right mental state for prayer or meditation.

Frankincense is a particularly good aid to the lungs, helping in cases of respiratory infection, nervous and allergic asthma, and chronic bronchitis.

ASTHMA RUB—CHILDREN 3–7
2 drops frankincense
3 drops lavender
2 drops geranium
Add to 1 tablespoon massage oil.

Massaging the chest area helps to open constricted lungs. Regular chest massage may prevent asthma attacks from occurring frequently. Asthmatics should test-smell essential oils to avoid individual allergic reactions.

ASTHMA RUB—SPASMODIC
3 drops frankincense
3 drops clary sage
2 drops peppermint

Add to 10 ml carrier oil, and massage on chest. Caution: Do not use on people with low blood pressure.

Geranium

Botanical Name: *Pelargonium graveolens*

Note: Middle **Odor Intensity:** High

KEY USES:
- Acne
- **Anxiety**
- Breast engorgement or congestion
- Bruises, broken capillaries
- Depression
- Diabetes
- Cellulite
- **Edema**
- Eczema
- **Hormone balance (PMS, menopause)**
- Insect repellant (mosquitoes, gnats)
- Kidney stones
- **Lymphatic stimulant**
- **Neuralgia (especially facial)**
- Skin care
- Urinary disorders
- Ulcers
- Wounds

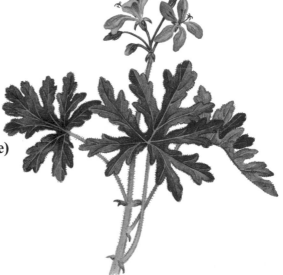

Aroma: Rose-like and sweet, with an earthy, mint-like undertone.

Blends well with: Clove, patchouli, sandalwood, neroli, jasmine, rose and all citrus, especially bergamot.

Part used: Leaves

Properties: Astringent, anti-inflammatory, antispasmodic, calming, diuretic, homeostatic, uplifting, vulnerary, tonic.

Emotional concerns: Geranium is useful in cases of nervous tension, stress, and anxiety.

Contraindications: Geranium can be an irritant to sensitive skin. It may cause restlessness or insomnia if used in the evening or if overused. Avoid long-term use if you have a history of estrogen-dependent cancers.

The essential oil of geranium has a flowery, rose-like fragrance. In fact, it is often used to adulterate rose oil. The essential oil of geranium comes from the pelargonium plant and should not be confused with the European genus of geranium, which includes crane's bill. Beware of falsified oils or oils from the wrong plant species.

Geranium is calming, balancing, and uplifting for depression. It is reputed to help with female hormone balance and is useful in easing PMS, engorgement of the breasts, night sweats, and hot flashes.

Geranium is helpful for general fatigue and tiredness. It is also good for many skin conditions, including bruises, fungal infections, wounds, dry skin, stretch marks, and cellulite.

WOUND HEALER
5 drops geranium
5 drops lavender
3 drops frankincense
1 tablespoon aloe vera gel

Mix and apply to the wound.

INSECT REPELLANT
4 drops thyme linalol
4 drops geranium
4 drops lavender
4 drops peppermint

Add to 2 tablespoons witch hazel and dilute in 4 oz. water. Spray on skin to deter insect bites.

Grapefruit, Pink

Botanical Name: *Citrus paradisi*

Note: Top   **Odor Intensity:** Medium

KEY USES:
- Anorexia
- **Cellulite**
- Circulation, poor
- **Depression**
- **Detoxification**
- Digestive problems
- Drug/alcohol withdrawal
- **Edema and fluid retention**
- Headache
- Jet lag
- Lymphatic congestion
- Obesity
- Weight loss

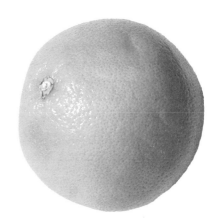

Aroma: Citrus, sweet, fresh, appealing.

Blends well with: All citrus, rosemary, lavender, thyme linalol, cinnamon, geranium.

Part used: Peel

Properties: Antidepressant, antiseptic, digestive, diuretic, stimulant, tonic.

Emotional concerns: Grapefruit is balancing to the emotions. It brightens dark, depressive moods, and it eases frustrations. Grapefruit provides a sense of lightness when everyday responsibilities seem too heavy.

Contraindications: Grapefruit has the shortest shelf life of the citrus essential oils but is the least photosensitizing. Because grapefruit is a potential skin irritant, it should not be used in large quantities in the bath.

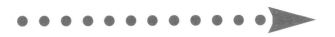

Grapefruit is valuable for conditions in which the body is not effectively eliminating toxins, including cellulite, fluid retention, and lymphatic congestion. Grapefruit stimulates the liver and gallbladder and helps regulate eating disorders. It is balancing for people who use overeating to calm nervous anxiety.

Grapefruit is helpful for general fatigue and tiredness. It is also good for many skin conditions, including bruises, fungal infections, wounds, dry skin, stretch marks, and cellulite.

CITRUS BODY POLISH
3 tablespoons jojoba oil
1 teaspoon NSP massage oil
3 tablespoons unscented castile soap
1 teaspoon Sunshine Concentrate
4 tablespoons fine sea salt
3 teaspoons coarse salt
25 drops bergamot
20 drops lemon
15 drops pink grapefruit

Gently stir together the soap and the oils. Add the salts and essential oils and blend with a wooden spoon. Transfer to a wide-mouthed container for easy scooping.

Apply this blend all over in the shower before turning on the water, paying special attention to rough areas such as elbows. Rinse. Enough for two applications.

Helichrysum

Botanical Name: *Helichrysum italicum*

Note: Middle   **Odor Intensity:** High

KEY USES:
- Allergies
- Arthritis
- **Bruises, burns, rashes**
- Chronic cough, whooping cough
- Dermatitis
- Detoxification
- **Eczema and psoriasis**
- Headaches and migraine
- Inflammation
- **Liver/spleen congestion**
- Meditation
- Muscle pain
- Nerve damage
- Nervous exhaustion
- Ringing in the ears
- **Scarring, wounds**

Aroma: Earthy, slightly floral, heady, powerful, hay-like.

Blends well with: Rose, lavender, Roman chamomile, geranium, clary sage.

Part used: Flowers

Properties: Anti-allergenic, anti-inflammatory, antitussive, antiseptic, cholagogue, cicatrizant, diuretic, expectorant, fungicidal, hepatic, nervine.

Emotional concerns: Helichrysum is relaxing and emotionally warming and opening, easing such emotions as frustration and irritability. According to Gabriel Mojay, the author of *Aromatherapy for Healing the Spirit*, helichrysum helps remove the most stubborn of wood emotions—jealousy, half-conscious anger, and bitterness of spirit.

Contraindications: Do not take internally.

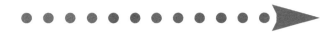

Helichrysum, also known as everlasting or immortelle, is native to the Mediterranean region. Like lavender, helichrysum stimulates the growth of new cells and is recommended for bruises, burns, and scars. Many claim that helichrysum can help with hearing loss and nerve damage, but these claims are as of yet scientifically unsubstantiated.

Helichrysum essential oil acts as a stimulant for the liver, gallbladder, and spleen. It aids in detoxification of the body, working especially through the lymph glands.

BLEND FOR BRUISES
3 drops helichrysum
3 drops lavender
2 drops geranium
2 drops thyme linalol
1 oz. carrier oil or lotion base

Mix the essential oils with the carrier oil or lotion. Apply to the bruise 3–4 times per day.

Jasmine

Botanical Name: *Jasminum officinale, Jasminum grandiflorum*

Note: Base **Odor Intensity:** High

KEY USES:
- **Aphrodisiac**
- Bronchial spasms
- Coughs, spasmodic
- Cramps, menstrual
- **Childbirth**
- Dry skin, dermatitis
- Impotence, frigidity (emotional)
- Milk production
- Post-partum depression
- **Perfume**
- Uterine spasms

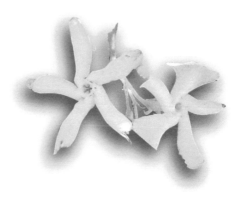

Fragrance: Deep, oriental, floral, sensuous.

Blends with: Sandalwood, rose, neroli, geranium.

Part used: Flowers

Properties: Analgesic, aphrodisiac, antidepressant, antispasmodic, carminative, cicatrizant, emollient, euphoric, expectorant, galactagogue, sedative, uterine tonic.

Emotional concerns: Hypersensitivity, lack of confidence, frigidity, impotence, post-partum depression, paranoia, fear.

Contraindications: Do not take internally. Beware of adulterated products. Do not use in the first four months of pregnancy. Use in low dilutions.

Jasmine essential oil has a rich, exotic smell, and it has been used as a perfume material for centuries. Louis XIV reportedly slept in jasmine-scented sheets. Jasmine is also a powerful aphrodisiac, and is reputed to help with both impotence and frigidity. It may be that jasmine has pheromone-like qualities, as it is in some ways chemically similar to pheromone-containing human perspiration (Wilson, 56).

Jasmine is helpful during childbirth; in small amounts it can reduce pain and stimulate uterine contractions (Walji, 57). It may also help to stimulate milk production after delivery.

Jasmine oil, like rose, is costly to produce. Jasmine flowers are delicate and must be picked by hand to prevent damage. Due to changes in the plant's chemistry, the aroma of jasmine becomes more intense at night (Davis, 173). For this reason, jasmine must be gathered before daylight, which increases labor costs. Due to its remarkable nocturnal fragrance, the people of India call jasmine "Queen of the Night."

LUXURIOUS BODY POWDER
5 drops sandalwood
2 drops jasmine
2 drops grapefruit
3 drops bergamot
1/2 cup cornstarch

SELF CONFIDENCE ROLL-ON
1 drop jasmine
1 drop rose
1 drops ylang ylang
3 drops thyme linalol
10 ml of carrier oil

Combine and put in roll-on bottle. Use throughout the day as a perfume; apply to pulse points.

Lavender

Botanical Name: *Lavandula angustifolia*

Note: Middle   **Odor Intensity:** Medium

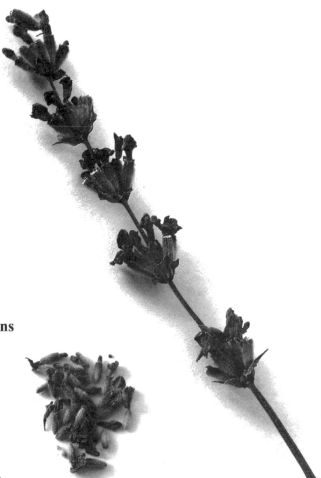

KEY USES:
- Acne
- Anger
- **Anxiety**
- **Bruises, burns, sunburn, cuts**
- Convulsions
- Eczema and psoriasis
- **Hair loss**
- **Headache and migraine**
- Hiccups
- Hypertension
- **Infection**
- **Insect bites**
- Insect repellent
- **Insomnia**
- **Inflammation**
- Leukorrhea
- Muscle spasms
- **Pain—arthritic, strains, sprains**
- Palpitations
- Rash, itchy skin
- Scabies
- Scars
- Vaginitis
- **Wounds**

Aroma: Floral and herbaceous, clean.

Blends well with: Most essential oils, especially geranium, clary sage, pine, thyme, peppermint and all citrus.

Part used: Leaves and flowers

Properties: Antidepressant, anti-inflammatory, antiseptic, aphrodisiac, astringent, antivenom, emmenagogue, hemostatic, sedative, tonic.

Emotional concerns: Lavender is very balancing and calming to the nervous system and can soothe states of anxiety, irritability, anger, frustration, and compulsion. Lavender may be helpful in cases of manic depression.

Contraindications: Use with caution during pregnancy. Be sure to use only true lavender, (*Lavandula angustifolia*). Other types of lavender have different properties and stronger contraindications.

Lavender is one of the most useful of all essential oils. It is perhaps most famous for its ability to accelerate the healing of wounds and burns. Lavender is also useful for coughs, colds, and sore throats. It is an effective relaxant and sedative and may be useful in cases of insomnia and nightmares.

Lavender essential oil is reputed to help with migraine headaches, and it is often used in skin care products due to its healing, soothing, and moisturizing properties. The name "lavender" may have come from the Latin word *lavare*, which means "to wash," because the Romans frequently used fragrant lavender in their bath waters.

Lemon

Botanical Name: *Citrus limonum*

Note: Top   **Odor Intensity:** Low

KEY USES:
- Arteriosclerosis
- Arthritis
- **Cellulite, cellular congestion**
- **Colds and flu**
- **Depression**
- Indigestion
- Infections
- Gallstones and urinary stones
- Gastric hyperacidity
- **Hypertension**
- Jet lag
- Liver congestion
- Varicose veins
- Warts

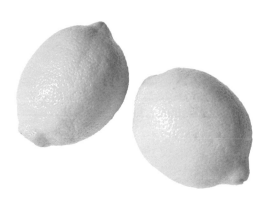

Aroma: Clean, fresh, citrus, penetrating.

Blends well with: lavender, ylang ylang, all other citrus, geranium, chamomile, eucalyptus, rose, thyme.

Part used: Peel

Properties: Antiseptic, anti-toxic, antiviral, bactericidal, digestive, diuretic, fungicidal, stimulant, stomachic, tonic.

Emotional concerns: Lemon is uplifting and rejuvenating. It can clear thinking and dispel sluggishness.

Contraindications: Lemon has a short shelf life. Old oil used on the skin may cause an allergic reaction. Lemon is photosensitizing, so avoid sunlight and tanning beds after application. Use only in low concentrations for all dermal applications and baths.

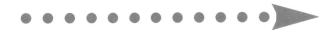

The lemon tree originated in Southeast Asia but is now grown extensively in hot climates around the world, particularly in California and the Mediterranean. The Greeks and Romans used lemon peel as an insect repellant. By the late 17th century, Europeans were using lemon as a blood purifier and digestive.

Lemon is effective in treating infections of all kinds and is believed to increase white blood cell activity. Lemon is tonifying to the circulatory and digestive systems and helps counteract acidity in the body.

COLDS
3 drops rosemary
2 drops peppermint
2 drops eucalyptus
3 drops lemon

Combine essential oils in an amber glass bottle.
Use 3–4 drops in a steam inhalation.

ANTISEPTIC SPRAY FOR THE HOME
10 drops lemon
3 drops thyme linalol
8 oz. distilled water
2 tablespoons alcohol

Add lemon to alcohol in a glass spray bottle. Add water. Shake before using.

Mandarin, Green or Red

Botanical Name: *Citrus reticulata*

Note: Top

Odor Intensity: Low (green) to Medium-High (red)

KEY USES:
- Acne
- Cellulite
- **Children's concerns**
- Dyspepsia
- Fluid retention
- **Hiccups**
- **Indigestion**
- **Insomnia**
- Intestinal problems
- Nervous tension
- Oily skin
- **Restlessness**
- **Stretch marks**
- Scars

Aroma: Fresh, citrus, lively.

Blends well with: Bergamot, cinnamon, clove, lavender, sandalwood.

Part used: Peel

Properties: Antiseptic, antispasmodic, carminative, digestive, diuretic (mild), sedative, tonic.

Emotional concerns: Stress, tension, moodiness, shock.

Contraindications: Photosensitizing; do not use on skin prior to sun exposure.

Like other quality citrus essential oils, mandarin is obtained by cold expression of the peel of the fruit. The result is an essential oil that has a sweet citrus aroma. Green mandarin tends to have a softer, more floral aroma, while the red mandarin's aroma is more pungent.

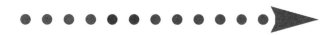

French aromatherapists consider mandarin to be one of the safest essential oils. Hence, it is used in children's remedies and by pregnant women and the elderly. It is often used for hiccups and to soothe indigestion. It may also support the liver. Like all citrus oils, mandarin is photosensitizing, which means that topical use may cause skin to burn more quickly and more deeply in sunlight or from tanning beds.

MANDARIN OILY SKIN TONER

6 ounces distilled water
3 drops mandarin
2 drops lemon
1 tablespoon witch hazel

Combine ingredients in a glass bottle. Shake mixture before use. This will have a shelf life of about one month.

For an even more natural toner, make an infusion of 1 heaping tablespoon of dried witch hazel herb in 1 cup of boiling water. Allow the mixture to steep for 10 minutes, then strain. Substitute the infusion for the distilled water and the prepared witch hazel in the above recipe.

STRETCH MARK PREVENTION

6 drops mandarin
4 drops neroli
2 drops geranium or 3 drops lavender
1 teaspoon each fresh flaxseed oil, fresh hazelnut oil, fresh rose hip seed oil
1 tablespoon of quality base oil such as wheat germ
1 Vitamin E capsule, cut open and added to mixture
1 ounce cocoa butter

Melt cocoa butter slowly over low heat in a small, stainless steel pan. Remove from heat and stir in the vegetable oils and vitamin E. Add the essential oils last, as the mixture is cooling.

High-quality carrier oils turn rancid very quickly and should be stored in the refrigerator. You can find flax seed oil in the refrigerated section of your health food store. If you cannot locate the rose hip seed oil or hazelnut oil, the recipe will still be effective. Instead, increase the base oil to 1 1/2 tablespoons.

Marjoram, Sweet

Botanical Name: *Origanum majorana*

Note: Middle   **Odor Intensity:** Medium

KEY USES:

- **Aches and pains**
- Amenorrhea
- Asthma
- Bronchitis
- Colds
- Colic
- Constipation
- Coughs
- Dyspepsia
- High blood pressure
- **Insomnia**
- **Joints, stiff**
- Leucorrhea
- Migraines
- Mouth ulcers
- **Muscle cramps**
- Nervous tension
- Painful menstruation
- Palpitations
- Rheumatism

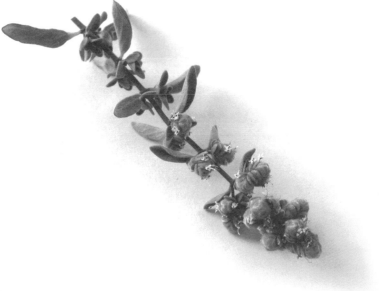

Aroma: Warm, woody, camphoraceous, green, nutty.

Blends well with: Lavender, bergamot, neroli, rosemary, tea tree, clary sage, geranium.

Parts used: Leaves

Properties: Anaphrodisiac, analgesic, antiseptic, antispasmodic, digestive, expectorant, hypotensive, laxative, nervine, restorative, sedative, tonic.

Emotional concerns: Loneliness, debility, insomnia, agitation, anguish, obsession, nervous tension.

Contraindications: Large amounts may cause drowsiness or dull the senses to the point of stupefaction. Do not use during pregnancy. May decrease sexual desire.

In ancient times, marjoram was believed to increase lifespan. Dioscorides recommended it for nervous disorders. Ancient Greek physicians used marjoram to treat rheumatism and muscle spasms. During the Renaissance, this marvelous herb was used for jaundice and chest infections (Walji, 110–111). Culpepper says marjoram herb "helpeth all diseases of the chest which hinder the breathing," and it is "comforting in cold diseases of the head, stomach, sinews and other parts…" (Culpepper, 227).

Marjoram is a wonderful sedative, a first choice for insomnia, nervous tension or anguish. It relieves muscle pain, being both analgesic and antispasmodic. A rub with marjoram after strenuous exercise is an excellent choice.

Marjoram is useful for colds and coughs, because it helps kill bacteria and aid the body in expelling mucus from the lungs. It also soothes the spasms often associated with cough.

DAYTIME AFTER EXERCISE MUSCLE RELIEF RUB
5 drops marjoram
4 drops rosemary
3 drops eucalyptus
2 drops peppermint
1 drop thyme
1/2 ounce carrier oil or aloe vera gel

NIGHTTIME MUSCLE RELIEF CREAM
5 drops marjoram
4 drops lavender
2 drop Roman chamomile
2 drops ylang ylang

Combine ingredients in 1/2 ounce of a cream-base lotion, such as self heal cream or Healing AC cream.

OFF TO SLEEP
3 drops marjoram
3 drops neroli
3 drops lavender

Use in a nebulizing diffuser or plug-in wall diffuser.

Myrrh

Botanical Name: *Commiphora myrrha*

Note: Base **Odor Intensity:** High

KEY USES:
- Aging or wrinkled skin
- Athlete's foot
- Bronchitis
- Colds
- **Coughs with thick mucus**
- **Cracked, chapped, or mature skin**
- **Cuts, sores, skin ulcers, bedsores**
- **Gingivitis**
- **Tooth, gum, and mouth infections**
- Sore throat/laryngitis
- Thrush
- Wound healing

Aroma: Smokey and resinous

Blends well with: Geranium, frankincense, rose

Part used: Resin

Properties: Antifungal, anti-inflammatory, antiseptic, fungicidal, expectorant, sedative, vulnerary.

Emotional concerns: Myrrh enhances spiritual connections and is calming and reassuring. It is also good for emotional confusion, fear, and hysteria.

Contraindications: Myrrh may be contraindicated in cases of low blood sugar. Avoid it during pregnancy, and use it in moderation.

Myrrh has a long history of use in religious ceremonies as incense. Ancient Egyptians also used it as an embalming agent. Myrrh was one of the three gifts of the Magi, along with frankincense and gold. Jesus was anointed with myrrh after his death. Ancient texts refer to the power of myrrh to hasten labor and treat rotten teeth.

Myrrh is helpful for eliminating excess thick mucous.

INHALATION FOR THICK MUCOUS
4 drops myrrh
3 drops eucalyptus
2 drops thyme
1-2 drops tea tree

Drop essential oils into a bowl of almost boiling water. Cover head with a towel and carefully inhale vapors deeply for five minutes. Repeat three times a day for five days, or until condition clears.

Neroli

Botanical Name: *Citrus aurantium var amara*

Note: Middle to Base   **Odor Intensity:** Medium

KEY USES:
- Anxiety
- **Childbirth**
- **Circulation**
- Dry, irritated skin
- Hemorrhoids
- **High blood pressure**
- Hysteria
- **Insomnia**
- Intestinal spasms
- Irritability
- Frigidity
- Mature skin
- **Palpitations**
- **Perfume**
- PMS
- Post-partum depression
- Rapid heart beat
- Scarring
- Shock
- Skin—all types
- Stress
- **Stretch marks**
- **Tachycardia**
- Varicose veins

Aroma: Sweet, citrus, heady with bitter undertone.

Blends well with: All citrus, lavender, rose, jasmine, chamomile.

Parts used: Flowers

Properties: Antiseptic, antidepressant, antispasmodic, anti-toxic, aphrodisiac, carminative, deodorant, euphoric, hypnotic, sedative, tonic, tranquilizing.

Emotional concerns: Neroli is useful for states such as shock or hysteria. It may be helpful for post-partum depression, irritability and sadness.

Contraindications: Do not confuse this oil with niaouli oil, a variety of tea tree.

The essential oil of neroli is distilled from the fresh-picked flowers of the orange tree, making it a citrus family member. Neroli is one of the most expensive and precious of the essential oils. One ton of hand-picked blossoms produces only one quart of essential oil. The best quality neroli oil comes from the bitter orange tree, which is cultivated for its perfume.

Neroli has powerful psychological properties. It helps relieve the strain of long-term tension, and it is a wonderful natural aid for insomnia. Neroli also helps to regulate heart rhythm and to lower blood pressure.

SOFT SKIN
2 drops neroli
1 drop Roman chamomile
1 drop rose
4 drops bergamot
2 capsules vitamin E, opened
1 ounce massage oil with borage

Mix all ingredients and use on skin after showering.

HIGH BLOOD PRESSURE
3 drop neroli
2 drops ylang ylang
4 drops lemon
1 drop lavender

Place in nebulizing diffuser. Turn on for several minutes to inhale aroma. Or place the mixture on the cotton pad of an aromaball to diffuse gently throughout the day.

PALPITATIONS/TACHYCARDIA ROLL-ON BLEND
2 drops neroli
1 drop rose
2 drops ylang ylang

Mix with 10 ml massage oil in roll-on bottle. Roll onto pulse point on wrists several times per day; inhale aroma directly throughout the day.

Oregano

Botanical Name: *Origanum vulgare and Origanum Compactum*

Note: Middle   **Odor Intensity:** Medium

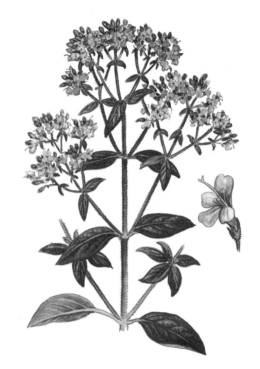

KEY USES:
- Amenorrhea
- **Arthritis**
- Asthma
- **Bronchitis (chronic)**
- **Candida**
- Cellulite
- Colds and flu
- Constipation
- Cough—tickling and whooping
- Constipation
- Digestion, sluggish
- Expectorant
- Lice
- Parasites
- Respiratory infection (tuberculosis)
- **Rheumatism**
- Warts

Aroma: Pungent, hot, earthy and spicy.

Blends well with: Lemon, bergamot, lavender, rose, pine, geranium, sandalwood.

Parts used: Leaves

Properties: Analgesic, antiseptic, antispasmodic, carminative, stomachic, expectorant, emmenagogue, antirheumatic.

Contraindications: Avoid prolonged internal use. May be irritating to the skin and cause contact dermatitis. Always dilute well before applying to the skin. Do not use during pregnancy or on children under age 5. Blend oregano with mild essential oils such as lavender before diffusing. Excessive amounts of diffused oregano will cause eye and throat irritation.

Undiluted oregano can be very irritating to the skin. Use only in dilution with vegetable oil or lotion. Be especially careful on hypersensitive skin, damaged skin, aged skin and with children.

Oregano is a strong antimicrobial oil and is generally a good choice for fighting colds. It also eases the pain of arthritis. However, oregano is a skin irritant and should be used with caution. Do not confuse *Origanum vulgare ssp compactum* with the more gentle essential oil of marjorum, *Origanum majorana*.

Patchouli

Botanical Name: *Pogostemon patchouli*

Note: Base **Odor Intensity:** High

KEY USES:
- Athlete's foot
- Abscesses
- Cold sores
- **Dry, cracked skin**
- **Eczema**
- Enlarged pores
- Fungal infections
- Hemorrhoids
- Impotence
- Scars
- Wounds, weeping sores

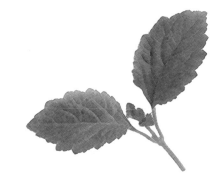

Aroma: Deep, earthy, intense, musty.

Blends well with: Geranium, bergamot, grapefruit, lavender, frankincense, rose, sandalwood, pine.

Aroma: Sweet, citrus, heady with bitter undertone.

Parts used: Leaves

Properties: Anti-inflammatory, antidepressant, aphrodisiac, fungicide, insecticide, sedative, tonic.

Emotional concerns: Patchouli is grounding and calming and helps with apathy, anorexia, and anxiety.

Contraindications: Use with moderation.

The fragrance of patchouli is deep, warm, and distinct. Patchouli leaves are aged before the distillation process, which helps to impart richness into the smell of this essential oil. As patchouli essential oil ages, its smell continues to improve and deepen. Patchouli helps to rejuvenate skin, so it is a good choice for aging skin and cracked, dry skin. It is also helpful for eczema, acne, and athlete's foot. Think of it as a remedy for whenever the skin is split, cracked, or purulent. Patchouli is antifungal and antiseptic, and is an excellent insect repellant, especially for wool moths.

CRACKED AND CALLOUSED HEELS

2 drops patchouli
2 lavender
1/2 teaspoon healing lotion base

Combine lotion and patchouli. Apply liberally to the heels. Cover with cotton socks overnight. Repeat for several nights.

Peppermint

Botanical Name: *Mentha piperita*

Note: Top   **Odor Intensity:** High

KEY USES:
- Asthma
- **Bad breath**
- **Bronchitis, chronic**
- **Colds and flu, dry cough**
- **Concentration, clarity, memory**
- **Decongestant**
- Fatigue, mental and physical
- Flatulence
- **Headache**
- **Gastrointestinal spasm**
- Gastrointestinal poisoning, diarrhea
- **Indigestion, heartburn, colic**
- Intestinal parasites
- **Irritable bowel syndrome**
- **Migraine**
- Muscle aches and pains
- **Nausea and vomiting**
- **Pain relief**
- Palpitations

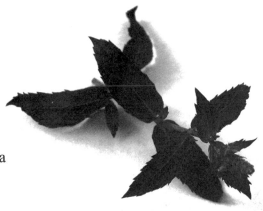

Aroma: Fresh, minty, earthy, sweet, penetrating, invigorating.

Blends well with: Lemon, rosemary, marjoram, eucalyptus, lavender.

Parts used: Leaves

Properties: Analgesic, antiseptic, anti-inflammatory, antispasmodic, expectorant, sudorific.

Emotional concerns: Peppermint helps with the assimilation and digestion of ideas. It stimulates and awakens the mind and refreshes the spirit.

Contraindications: Peppermint may counteract homeopathic remedies, and it may cause wakefulness in the evenings. Due to its cooling effect, do not rub peppermint over the whole body, and use with caution and only in diluted form in the bath.

RECIPE FOR DRY COUGH
5 drops peppermint
4 drops sandalwood
3 drops pine

Combine with 1 1/2 teaspoons aloe vera gel and rub onto chest. Or add to a bowl of almost boiling water and use as an inhalation.

RECIPE FOR GASTROINTESTINAL DISTRESS
2 drops peppermint
2 drops Roman chamomile
1 teaspoon carrier oil or lotion

Massage over affected area in a clockwise direction. The antispasmodic properties of peppermint oil will relieve the smooth muscles of the digestive tract, while its analgesic properties will ease pain. This combination of properties provides relief for colic, indigestion, vomiting, diarrhea, stomach pain, and intestinal cramps. The addition of Roman chamomile may augment the effect.

Pine

Botanical Name: *Pinus sylvestris*

Note: Middle   **Odor Intensity:** Medium

<u>KEY USES:</u>
- **Asthma**
- **Bronchitis**, laryngitis
- Colds
- **Deodorizer**
- Dysmenorrhea
- Fatigue
- **Flu**
- Hay fever
- **Respiratory infections** (pneumonia)
- Sinusitis

Native to Northern Europe and Russia, *Pinus sylvestris* is believed to be the only European pine to have survived the ice age. In Switzerland, pine needles are sometimes used to stuff mattresses as a way of treating rheumatic complaints. Pine is often recommended for lung and respiratory infection, for colds, and for disinfecting and deodorizing. Pine spritzed or diffused in a room is wonderful for eliminating odors.

Aroma: Clean, crisp, resinous, pungent.

Blends well with: Frankincense, lavender, lemon, patchouli, rosemary, peppermint, thyme, marjoram, bergamot.

Parts used: Needles

Properties: Antiseptic, antiviral, antirheumatic, deodorant, disinfectant, cholagogue, decongestant, diuretic, expectorant, tonic, stimulant.

Emotional concerns: Pine clears negative thoughts and helps with mental fatigue, self-esteem, and emotional weakness.

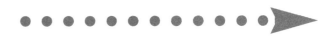

Contraindications: Those with a history of prostate cancer should avoid using pine. Pine may be a possible irritant to skin and kidneys. Do not use in large amounts in the bath.

LUNG INFECTION HEALING INHALATION
2 drops lavender
3 drops pine
3 drops thyme linalol
2 drops eucalyptus

Drop essential oils into a bowl of almost boiling water. Cover head with a towel and carefully inhale vapors deeply for five minutes. Repeat three times daily for 10 days.

Rose

Botanical Name: *Rosa damascena*

Note: Middle   **Odor Intensity:** Very High

<u>**KEY USES:**</u>
- Aging, delicate skin
- **Aphrodisiac**
- Broken capillaries
- Depression
- Eczema
- **Grief**
- Liver problems
- **Menopause**
- PMS
- Uterine tonic

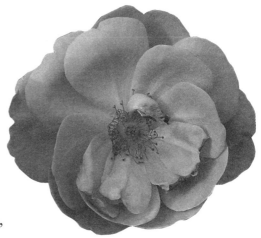

Aroma: Sweet and floral with complex undertones.

Blends well with: Lemon, bergamot, clary sage, geranium, lavender, Roman chamomile, sandalwood, ylang ylang, jasmine.

Parts used: Flowers

Properties: Antidepressant, anti-inflammatory, antiseptic, aphrodisiac, astringent, emmenagogue, hemostatic, sedative, tonic.

Emotional concerns: Rose is useful in treating depression, emotional coldness, sadness, anger, stress, bereavement, nervous tension, and insomnia.

Contraindications: Use with caution during pregnancy. Beware of adulteration with Geranium essential oil.

Perhaps no other flower has more romantic symbolism than the rose. Its fragrance has inspired poets and lovers since ancient times.

Rose essential oil has been used in Persia for hundreds of years. In fact, the Persians were the first to distill the essential oil of rose. The Gallica rose—often referred to as the Damask rose—is the variety most highly valued. The essential oil produced from roses in Bulgaria's Kanzanlik Valley are considered the best and most fragrant. One acre of land yields three tons of Damask roses, which in turn yield only two liters of essential oil after distillation (Howe, 86).

Turkey also produces essential oil of rose. It is less expensive and considered to be less desirable, but it still has a beautiful smell.

THREAD VEINS AND TENDER SKIN
2 drops rose
3 drops lavender
4 teaspoons witch hazel
2 oz. rose water

Combine and apply to the cheeks twice a day. Also use as a cool compress.

Rosemary

Botanical Name: *Rosemarinus officinalis*

Note: Middle **Odor Intensity:** High

KEY USES:
- **Arthritis and rheumatism**
- Asthma
- **Bronchitis**
- Cellulite
- **Circulation, poor**
- **Colds, cough and flu**
- **Constipation**
- Dysmenorrhea
- Edema, water retention
- Hair loss, dandruff
- **Headache**
- Hypotension
- Intestinal infections
- Lice, scabies
- Lymphatic congestion
- **Memory loss, mental fatigue**
- Migraine
- Muscle soreness
- **Stimulant**
- Whooping cough

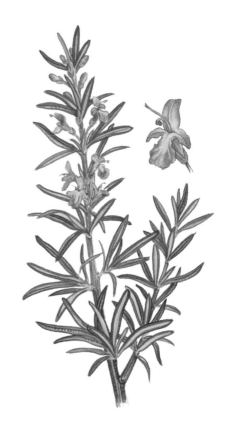

Aroma: Camphoraceous, penetrating, fresh.

Blends well with: Grapefruit, bergamot, lavender, peppermint, pine, geranium, tea tree, thyme.

Parts used: Leaves and twigs

Properties: Antiseptic, analgesic, antirheumatic, astringent, antispasmodic, carminative, cephalic, diaphoretic, digestive, decongestant, diuretic, emmenagogue, hypertensive, parasiticide, stimulant, tonic.

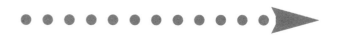

Emotional concerns: Rosemary is useful in cases of mental fatigue, lethargy, and forgetfulness. It promotes mental clarity and clears the mind of doubt and confusion.

Contraindications: Avoid use during pregnancy or on those with a history of high blood pressure or epilepsy. Do not use on sensitive or damaged skin. Rosemary may have antifertility effects, preventing egg implantation. Large quantities of ingested rosemary oil may cause intestinal irritation and renal damage (Fetrow, 554–555).

Rosemary is energizing. It stimulates the central nervous system, aids the lymphatic system by eliminating wastes from the body, and is a good choice for edema and cellulite. In the bath or as a massage, rosemary helps to improve circulation. It also improves circulation in the scalp and can be used in cases of dandruff and hair loss.

Rosemary is also helpful for muscle pains and rheumatism. For rheumatism, use in a friction rub with alcohol, and for muscle pains use in a friction rub with olive oil or other massage oil.

SCALP TREATMENT FOR HAIR LOSS
1 tablespoon jojoba oil
2 teaspoons massage oil
8 drops lavender
5 drops clary sage
3 drops rosemary
3 drops grapefruit or 3 drops ylang ylang

Blend. Warm the mixture in your hands or in warm water before application. Massage a few drops into the scalp and leave overnight to be absorbed. Apply 3–4 times weekly.

Sandalwood

Botanical Name: *Santalum album*

Note: Base   **Odor Intensity:** Medium

KEY USES:
- **Aphrodisiac**
- **Bladder infection, cystitis**
- **Bronchitis, persistent**
- **Calming and grounding**
- Cough, dry
- Cracked skin
- Diarrhea
- Eczema
- Kidney infections
- Impotence
- **Spiritual aid**
- Urinary tract problems

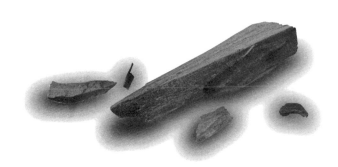

Aroma: Woody, deep, lasting, musky, sweet, balsamic.

Blends well with: Chamomile, patchouli, geranium, bergamot, jasmine, frankincense, rose, ylang ylang.

Parts used: Heartwood

Properties: Antifungal, antiphlogistic, antiseptic, antispasmodic, aphrodisiac, astringent, decongestant, diuretic, emollient, expectorant, insecticide, sedative, tonic.

Emotional concerns: Sandalwood can be helpful with obsession and materialism.

Contraindications: Use with moderation.

Sandalwood is one of the oldest known sources of perfume and incense. It has been used in India since ancient times for religious rituals, and temples have been built of sandalwood. As a powerful meditation and prayer aid, it helps the mind set aside mental chatter and create the right mood for worship.

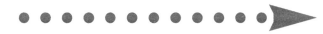

Medicinal uses of sandalwood are mentioned in old Sandkrit and Chinese manuscripts. In Chinese medicine, it is used to treat stomachache, vomiting, and gonorrhea. In Ayurvedic medicine, sandalwood is used for urinary and respiratory tract infections, skin inflammations, abscesses, and tumors.

Sandalwood essence is derived from the heartwood of the sandalwood tree. The trees grow very slowly, reaching maturity in 40 to 50 years. Cut sandalwood is left on the forest floor until the outer wood is eaten away by ants, leaving only the heartwood, which the ants will not attack. Sandalwood essential oil is steam-distilled from this heartwood.

RELAXING BATH
5–6 drops sandalwood
2–3 drops Roman chamomile

Combine essential oils with 1 teaspoon of honey. Add honey and oil mixture to running bath water.

Tea Tree

Botanical Name: *Melaleuca alternifolia*

Note: Top   **Odor Intensity:** Very High

KEY USES:

- Abscesses
- **Acne**
- Air purifier
- Asthma
- Athlete's foot
- **Burns and bruises**
- Candida
- **Colds and flu**
- **Coughs and catarrh**
- **Cold sores, mouth ulcers**
- Cuts, burns, bites
- Cystitis, itching
- Dandruff
- Herpes, chicken pox
- Lice
- **Nail infections**
- Parasites
- **Respiratory infections**
- Ringworm
- Sinusitis
- Tonsillitis
- Vaginitis
- Warts
- Wound healing

Aroma: Pungent, aggressive, camphor-like, clean.

Blends well with: Lavender, geranium, pine, thyme, clary sage, grapefruit, bergamot.

Parts used: Leaves

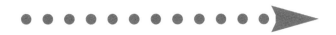

Properties: Antibiotic, antibacterial, antifungal, antiseptic, antiviral, decongestant, deodorant, diaphoretic, antifungal, expectorant, immune stimulant, antiparasitic, vermifuge, vulnerary.

Emotional concerns: Tea tree oil is good for cases of depression and low self-esteem.

Contraindications: Tea tree may be a possible irritant to sensitive skin despite its reputation as safe for neat application.

The tea tree is a small Australian tree related to the eucalyptus tree. The essential oil is distilled from the tree's leaves, which are small and needle-like.

Tea tree essential oil is a strong antifungal and antibacterial oil but is generally mild to the skin. In damp climates, tea tree oil has been used in air ventilation systems to reduce mold growth.

Thyme Linalol

Botanical Name: *Thymus vulgaris ct. linalol*

Note: Middle   **Odor Intensity:** Medium

KEY USES:

- **Asthma**
- Amenorrhea
- Athlete's foot
- Bronchitis
- Boils, cuts, sores
- **Colds and flu**
- Fatigue, mental and physical
- Fever
- Hypotension
- **Infections—skin, intestines**
- Infectious diseases
- Leukorrhea
- Lymphatic cleanser
- **Parasites**
- Rheumatism
- Sinusitis
- Sore throat
- **Tonsillitis**
- **Whooping cough, convulsive cough**

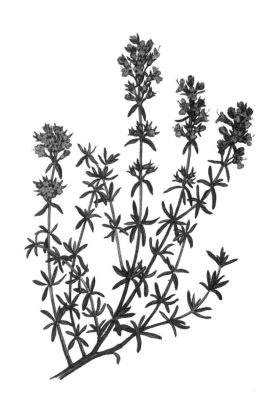

Aroma: Fresh, herbaceous, penetrating, green.

Blends well with: Lavender, bergamot, marjoram, pine, geranium, lemon, peppermint.

Parts used: Leaves and stem

Properties: Antiseptic, antispasmodic, antitussive, antivenomous, antiputrefactive, cicatrizing, emmenagogue, expectorant, hypertensive, parasidicide, sudorific, vermifuge.

Emotional concerns: Thyme linalol can be helpful in cases of low self-esteem, mental instability, and melancholy.

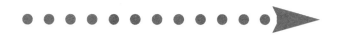

Contraindications: Do not use during pregnancy or on those with epileptic conditions, hyperthyroidism, or high blood pressure.

Thyme may have been used as long ago as 3500 B.C. by the Sumarians. The Romans believed that thyme imbued bravery, and soldiers would be sent bath waters with thyme before marching to battle. Hildegarde of Bingen suggested using thyme for body lice, plague, leprosy, and paralysis.

The species *Thymus vulgaris* produces eight different chemotypes. When thyme is grown at sea level, it is high in the phenol thymol, and is designated as *Thymus vulgaris ct. thymol*, or simply "thyme thymol." When thyme is grown in the mountains, it is high in the gentle alcohol linalol. The plant is referred to as *Thymus vulgaris ct. linalol* or simply "thyme linalol," or sometimes, "sweet thyme." Thyme linalol, due to the alcohol linalol, is also much more gentle to the skin than the other chemotypes. And unlike the other thyme chemotypes, it can be used on children and the elderly.

Ylang Ylang

Botanical Name: *Canaga odorata*

Note: Base   **Odor Intensity:** Medium

KEY USES:
- Acne
- Anger
- **Aphrodisiac**
- **Hypertension**
- **Intestinal infections**
- Impotence, frigidity
- **Palpitations, tachycardia**
- **Rapid breathing**
- Stress
- Uterine tonic

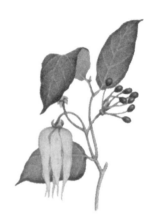

Aroma: Sweet, exotic, heavy, floral, rich, wet.

Blends well with: Sandalwood, jasmine, bergamot, clary sage, rose, patchouli.

Parts used: Flowers

Properties: Antidepressant, antiseptic, euphoric, hypotensive, nervine, sedative, tonic.

Emotional concerns: Ylang ylang is useful in treating anger, anxiety, panic, insomnia and low self-esteem.

Contraindications: Avoid use on damaged skin. Those with a history of low blood pressure or sleep apnea should also avoid using this oil. Use in moderation; high concentrations can induce headaches or nausea.

The ylang ylang tree originated in the Philippines but now grows throughout tropical Asia. The trees bear fragrant drooping yellow flowers, which are cultivated for the perfume trade. Ylang ylang may be purchased in several commercial grades, including extra, first, second, third, and complete. Beware of the less expensive canaga oil, which has an inferior scent.

9

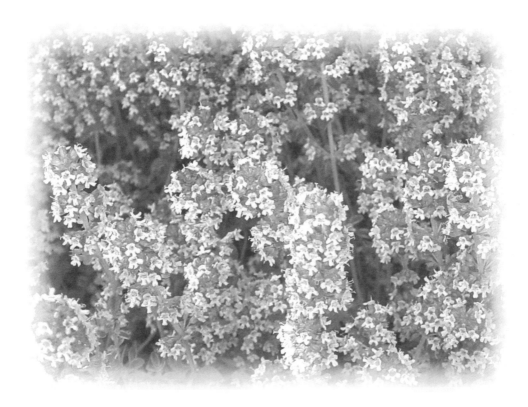

Aromatherapy and the Body Systems

The Digestive and Intestinal Systems

<u>KEY OILS:</u> **Peppermint, chamomile, clove, oregano, lemon**

Essential oils can provide tremendous aid to these systems. Essential oils can be used both externally and internally (with prudence). Results include instant relief from pain, cramping, indigestion and nausea.

THERAPEUTIC ACTIONS OF ESSENTIAL OILS ON THE DIGESTIVE AND INTESTINAL SYSTEMS

Anti-inflammatory—Reduces inflammation, irritation and pain. **Oils:** Chamomile, peppermint, lavender, marjoram

Antispasmodic—Reduces spasms and cramping. **Oils:** Chamomile, peppermint, lavender, marjoram

Antimicrobial—Reduces the growth of unwanted microorganisms such as bacteria or yeast. **Oils:** Oregano, lemon, bergamot, clove, thyme linalol

Digestive—Increases the secretion of digestive fluids and may improve digestion and appetite. **Oils:** Bergamot, grapefruit, peppermint, rosemary

Carminative—Causes expelling of gas from the intestines, aids nausea. **Oils:** Peppermint, clove, lemon

Cholagogue—Stimulates the gallbladder and improves the flow of bile. **Oils:** Lavender, peppermint

Hepatic—Affecting the liver, whether stimulating, toning or strengthening. **Oils:** Lemon, peppermint, rosemary, helichrysum

Stomachic—Tones or stimulates the stomach; aids nausea. **Oils:** Chamomile, bergamot, peppermint

Vermifuge—Destroys or expels intestinal worms. **Oils:** Cinnamon, clove, oregano, rosemary, lemon

Conditions and Therapeutic Treatments

CONDITION: Appetite Control
ESSENTIAL OILS: Pink grapefruit, bergamot
HERBS AND SUPPLEMENTS: Gymnema, blue-green algae, chromium, B-complex

Grapefruit is helpful in controlling comfort eating, while bergamot is helpful for compulsive eating (see anorexia).

CONDITION: Appetite Loss
ESSENTIAL OILS: Clove, rosemary, oregano
HERBS AND SUPPLEMENTS

Essential oils traditionally used for culinary purposes, such as clove or rosemary, can be used to stimulate the appetite. Inhale from a tissue, or directly from the bottle.

CONDITION: Bad Breath
ESSENTIAL OILS: Rosemary, peppermint, bergamot, thyme, clove, myrrh
HERBS AND SUPPLEMENTS: SAMe, intestinal and cellular cleanses, algin, chlorophyll, cysteine, digestive enzymes

> ### *Cinnamon Mint Mouthwash*
> 1/4 cup warm water
> 1 medium cinnamon stick, broken into small pieces
> 1/8 cup vodka
> 2 drops peppermint essential oil
> 1 drop clove essential oil (optional)

Heat the water to just under boiling. Add the cinnamon and allow mixture to cool. The cinnamon should infuse in the water overnight. After infusing, strain the water to remove the cinnamon pieces. Dissolve the peppermint and clove in the vodka. Add the cinnamon water to the vodka mixture and shake before using. Do not swallow.

CONDITION: Body Odor
ESSENTIAL OILS: Lemon, bergamot, thyme linalol, lavender, geranium
HERBS AND SUPPLEMENTS: SAMe, intestinal and cellular cleanses, algin, chlorophyll, cystine, digestive enzymes

> ### *Deodorant Spray 1*
> 2 drops each thyme, lemon, bergamot, lavender
> 1/4 teaspoon witch hazel
> 1/2 ounce distilled water

Pour ingredients into a glass misting bottle. Spray under arms as needed.

Deodorant Lotion

Use 1–2 drops of lavender neat under each arm. Or mix 2–3 drops of geranium in aloe vera gel or pau d'arco lotion and apply under arms. For extremely stressful days, try two drops thyme linalol and one drop of lemon mixed in pau d' arco lotion.

Deodorant Spray 2
1/2 ounce apple cider vinegar
3 ounces R.O. or distilled water
1 teaspoon witch hazel

30 drops of essential oils of your choice. Or use mine: 7 drops thyme, 3 drops geranium, 5 drops lavender, 3 drops peppermint, 4 drops lemon, 3 drops sandalwood, 2 drops clove, 3 drops tea tree.

Combine ingredients in a 4-ounce glass spray bottle. Spray under arms as needed.

CONDITION: **Candida**
ESSENTIAL OILS: Oregano, tea tree, thyme, bergamot, lavender, cinnamon, myrrh
HERBS AND SUPPLEMENTS: Noni juice, caprylic acid, olive leaf, garlic, acidophilus, bifidus, pau d'arco, olive oil, vitamin C, B-complex

The Candida Slide
1 drop oregano
2 drops tea tree
1 drop myrrh
1 drop cinnamon
2 teaspoons olive oil

Combine essential oils in olive oil. Use twice a day for 10 days. Take a break after 10 days to give your liver a rest.

CONDITION: **Constipation**

ESSENTIAL OILS: Marjoram, oregano, rosemary, neroli, peppermint
HERBS AND SUPPLEMENTS: Magnesium, cascara sagrada, whole leaf aloe juice

Constipation Rub 1
2 drops each peppermint and oregano
3 drops each rosemary and marjoram
1/2 ounce aloe vera gel

Rub on abdomen; cover with warm, damp cloth. Do this twice per day.

Constipation Rub 2

Rub 1 drop oregano neat into the sole of each foot. Concentrate on corresponding reflexology points.

CONDITION: Detoxification
ESSENTIAL OILS: Lemon, bergamot, grapefruit, helichrysum, thyme linalol
HERBS AND SUPPLEMENTS: Psyllium hulls, bentonite clay, activated charcoal, algin, vitamin C, B-vitamins, SAM-e, beets, lecithin, alfalfa, chlorophyll, green drinks

Detoxification Bath
3 drops lemon
3 drops bergamot
3 drops thyme linalol
1–2 drops helichrysum
1/2 cup hydrated bentonite
1/2 cup Epsom salts or sea salts or 1/4 cup ground kelp

First, dry brush the skin and rinse away the skin debris. Mix essential oils into salts. Add salts and clay to a warm running bath, soak for 15 to 20 minutes. Baths are extremely effective for removing toxins and soaking away aches and pains.

CONDITION: Diverticulosis

ESSENTIAL OILS: Bergamot, peppermint, rosemary, clove, chamomile
HERBS AND SUPPLEMENTS: Acidophilus and bifidus, aloe vera juice (whole leaf), flax seed oil or evening primrose oil, vitamin E, super antioxidant, bulk laxative, bromelain, slippery elm bark and broad-spectrum digestive enzymes. Herbs that soothe the nervous system and relax muscles such as chamomile and valerian may also help.

Regular use of essential oils can help ease the flatulence, cramping, inflammation and pain associated with this disease. Dietary changes are critical for the healing of diverticulosis. Check for food allergies and increase natural fiber in the diet.

Abdominal Rub
2 drops bergamot
2 drops peppermint
2 drops rosemary
1 drop clove
2 drops chamomile

Dilute in 15 ml carrier oil. Rub mixture on the abdomen twice daily.

CONDITION: Dysbiosis
ESSENTIAL OILS: Bergamot, oregano, thyme, lemon, rosemary
HERBS AND SUPPLEMENTS: Acidophilus and bifidus, whole leaf aloe vera, olive leaf

Recipe 1
1 drop bergamot
1 drop lemon
8 ounces RO or distilled water

Put essential oils in water. Shake bottle thoroughly before each sip.

Recipe 2
4 drops bergamot
2 drops thyme linalol
2 drops oregano
1/2 ounce massage oil or aloe vera gel

Mix together and massage into abdomen twice daily.

CONDITION: Hiccups

ESSENTIAL OILS: Mandarin
HERBS AND SUPPLEMENTS: Digestive enzymes

Hiccup Stopper
2 drops red mandarin
1 drop cinnamon leaf (not bark!)
1 teaspoon vegetable oil

Mix and drizzle down throat. The cinnamon leaf may be omitted if desired.

CONDITION: Indigestion
ESSENTIAL OILS: Peppermint, lemon
HERBS AND SUPPLEMENTS: Digestive enzymes, papaya tablets

Use 1 drop of peppermint internally to ease indigestion and stomach pain.

Peppermint Tea
1/2 teaspoon honey, added to mug first
1 drop each peppermint and grapefruit

Place honey in mug. Drop essential oils directly onto the honey and stir them together. Add hot water. The honey will emulsify the essential oils.

CONDITION: Irritable Bowel
ESSENTIAL OILS: Roman chamomile, peppermint
HERBS AND SUPPLEMENTS: Slippery elm bark, acidophilus and bifidus, calcium, magnesium, alfalfa, chamomile, aloe vera, l-glutamine, Super Antioxidant, STR-J, B-complex, valerian, turmeric, alpha lipoic acid.

Intestinal IBS Balancer
3 drops bergamot
2 drops Roman chamomile
2 drops peppermint
2 drops clary sage
2 drops thyme linalol

Dilute essential oils in 15 ml carrier oil or base lotion. Rub over intestinal area. This recipe will help with the cramps associated with IBS. It may also aid in clearing intestinal infections.

IBS Soother

Peppermint taken internally has been shown to reduce IBS. Use small amounts (1 to 2 drops) in 1 teaspoon of a carrier oil such as olive oil.

CONDITION: Parasites
ESSENTIAL OILS: Bergamot, chamomile, cinnamon, clove, eucalyptus, oregano, rosemary, tea tree, thyme

> ***Ascaris and Oxyuris:*** Eucalyptus, chamomile
> ***Hookworms:*** Thyme, clove
> ***Tapeworm:*** Thyme
> ***Roundworm:*** Chamomile, eucalyptus, thyme
> ***Pinworm/Threadworm:*** Chamomile, eucalyptus, lemon, thyme

HERBS AND SUPPLEMENTS: Noni juice, whole leaf aloe vera, Para-Cleanse, olive leaf, garlic, elecampane, artemesia, black walnut, anamu.

Parasite Rub
2 drops clove
1 drop cinnamon
1 drop oregano
4 drops thyme linalol
1 drop peppermint
1/2 to 1 ounce aloe vera gel or massage lotion,
   depending on skin sensitivity

Mix essential oils into aloe vera gel or massage lotion. Use more aloe or massage oil if you have sensitive skin. Do not use a synthetic lotion with mineral oil as it may impede absorption. Massage into stomach and abdomen and place warm towels over each application. Use this rub 2–3 times a day while you are on an herbal parasite cleanse. It really makes a difference! Be cautious with sensitive skin—do not overuse.

CONDITION: Nausea

ESSENTIAL OILS: Lemon, peppermint
HERBS AND SUPPLEMENTS: Ginger, papaya tablets, digestive enzymes, B-complex

Smell oils directly from the bottle. Also, take 1 drop of peppermint internally.

CONDITION: Spastic Colon
ESSENTIAL OILS: Roman chamomile, marjoram, bergamot, lavender
HERBS AND SUPPLEMENTS: Magnesium, Intestinal Soothe and Build, acidophilus, bifidus

> ### *Colon Calmer*
> 3 drops Roman chamomile
> 2 drops marjoram
> 2 drops bergamot
> 1 teaspoon massage oil

Combine ingredients and rub this concentrated, relaxing oil directly over the painful area, massaging from right to left along the colon. Cover with a hot, moist towel. I have seen this remedy soothe intestinal spasms in less than one minute.

CONDITION: Toothache

Place one drop of clove oil directly on the painful tooth. Use this remedy only on adults, and be aware that the clove will irritate the gum. Do not use on the elderly or people with fragile or painful gums.

The Circulatory System

<u>KEY OILS:</u> **Neroli, ylang ylang, lemon, lavender, rosemary, rose**

Essential oils can have a profound effect on the circulatory system. Just smelling the aroma of neroli can lower blood pressure, while the fragrance of ylang ylang may calm an over-rapid heart. It is easy to understand oils' effects on this system when you consider what a calming effect they have on the emotions and the body as a whole. The stress-relieving action of essential oils may help to lower heart rate and blood pressure. A full-body massage may be one of the best ways to use essential oils to prevent disorders of the circulatory system. A massage also assists the heart in delivering blood and oxygen to the body, especially the extremities.

THERAPEUTIC ACTIONS OF ESSENTIAL OILS ON THE CIRCULATORY SYSTEM	
Hypertensive—An agent that raises blood pressure. **Oils:** Rosemary, thyme linalol **Hypotensive**—An agent that lowers blood pressure. **Oils:** Neroli, lavender, ylang ylang, marjoram	**Nervine**—Soothing to the nervous system. **Oils:** Lavender, neroli, roman chamomile, mandarin **Astringent**—Tones the system, good for hemorrhoids and varicose veins. **Oils:** Lemon, geranium, grapefruit

Conditions and Therapeutic Treatments

CONDITION: Hemorrhoids
ESSENTIAL OILS: Geranium, lavender (pain), myrrh, Roman chamomile
HERBS AND SUPPLEMENTS: Garlic, slippery elm bark, white oak bark, Vari-Gone, soft bulk laxative with oat bran and psyllium, rutin, vitamin C, bioflavonoids, flax seed oil

Hemorrhoid Ointment
3 drops lavender
3 drops geranium
2 drops myrrh
2 drops Roman chamomile
1/2 ounce Golden Salve

Blend ingredients and rub onto the affected area. This ointment will reduce swelling and irritation, and reduce the chance of infection.

CONDITION: High Blood Pressure
ESSENTIAL OILS: Neroli, lavender, ylang ylang, marjoram, Roman chamomile, clary sage
HERBS AND SUPPLEMENTS: Magnesium, garlic, capsicum, parsley, coenzyme Q10, B-complex, flax seed oil or omega-3 fatty acids, herbal stress formula, passion flower, calcium, l-glutamine, lecithin, vitamin E, reishi mushroom, herbal potassium

High Blood Pressure Massage Oil
2 drops ylang ylang
3 drops lemon
2 drops lavender
2 drops marjoram
2 drops clary sage
15 ml massage oil

Use for a full body massage.

Hypertension Calming Pulse Point Roll-on
1 drop neroli
3 drops bergamot
1–3 drops lavender
1–2 drops ylang ylang or marjoram

Mix with 10 ml massage oil in roll-on bottle. Roll onto pulse point on wrists several times per day, and bring the aroma to your nose throughout the day.

CONDITION: Low Blood Pressure
ESSENTIAL OILS: Rosemary, Thyme linalol, eucalyptus, pine
HERBS AND SUPPLEMENTS: Capsicum, dandelion, ginkgo, licorice, ginseng

Brisk Local Massage
3 drops rosemary
2 drops pine
1 drop oregano or cinnamon leaf
1 teaspoon massage oil or aloe vera gel

Blend massage oils and essential oils. Use for a brisk local massage of chest or extremities.

CONDITION: Poor Circulation
ESSENTIAL OILS: Peppermint, Tei Fu, rosemary, bergamot, eucalyptus, lemon, pine, thyme linalol, lavender, marjoram, rose
HERBS AND SUPPLEMENTS: Capsicum, vitamin chelation formula

Circulation Rub 1
3 drops thyme linalol
2 drops rosemary
1 drop rose
1 drop geranium

Add to 1 ounce massage oil and rub into extremities.

Cooling Circulation Rub
3 drops peppermint
4 drops eucalyptus
3 drops lavender

Add to 1/2 ounce massage oil and rub into extremities.

CONDITION: Palpitations/Tachycardia
ESSENTIAL OILS: Ylang ylang, neroli, rose
HERBS AND SUPPLEMENTS: B-complex, magnesium, herbal stress blend, hawthorn berry, l-carnitine, co-Q10

Palpitations Roll-on Blend
2 drops neroli
1 drop rose
1–2 drops ylang ylang or 3 drops lavender

Mix with 10 ml massage oil in roll-on bottle. Roll onto pulse point on wrists several times per day, and bring aroma to your nose throughout the day.

CONDITION: **Varicose Veins**
ESSENTIAL OILS: Lemon, rose, frankincense, geranium
HERBS AND SUPPLEMENTS: Proanthocyanidins (Grapine, pycnogenol), Vari-Gone, lecithin, vitamin C with bioflavonoids, rutin, horse chestnut, butcher's broom, vitamin E, co-Q10, psyllium hulls, glutathione, garlic

Varicose Vein Lotion
2 drops Cellutone
1 drops lemon
1 drop bergamot
1 drop rose (optional)
1 teaspoon Varigone lotion

Combine lotion with oils in the palm of your hand. Apply mixture gently to affected area, stroking lightly up towards the heart. Use daily.

The Respiratory System

<u>KEY OILS:</u> **Eucalyptus, peppermint, frankincense**

Observing the effects of essential oils on the respiratory system brings great understanding. Essential oils can open the lungs, deepen breathing and greatly help in overcoming difficult chest infections. Essential oils can also be used to kill ambient mold particles and odors in the air, making it more pleasant to breathe. Polluted air may be one of the biggest strains on the respiratory system. Pollution and cigarette smoke can cause the cilia that line the respiratory tract to die, and deposit deadly residues on our lung tissues.

THERAPEUTIC ACTIONS OF ESSENTIAL OILS ON THE RESPIRATORY SYSTEM	
Antispasmodics—Relax spasms of the respiratory tract; especially important with colds, nagging coughs and asthma. **Oils:** Clary sage, Roman chamomile, marjoram **Antimicrobials**—Oils that effectively kill bacteria, viruses and fungi. **Oils:** Thyme linalol, cinnamon leaf, clove, lemon, eucalyptus, tea tree, oregano, frankincense, lavender	**Expectorants**—Promote the expulsion of mucus. **Oils:** Peppermint, pine, eucalyptus **Pulmonary**—Relating to the lungs; in this case opening or deepening the breathing. **Oils:** Frankincense, peppermint

Conditions and Therapeutic Treatments

CONDITION: Asthma
ESSENTIAL OILS: Peppermint, clary sage, frankincense, lavender, marjoram, myrrh, rosemary, thyme linalol
HERBS AND SUPPLEMENTS: Vitamin C, vitamin E, proanthocyanidins (pycnogenol and Grapine), B-complex, lobelia, yerba santa

Check for food allergies and remove preservatives and other chemicals from your diet. Proanthocyanidins act as natural antihistamines. Use lobelia to relax the lungs in acute attacks.

Many different aromatherapy recipes for asthma exist. Use caution with your oil choice when helping people with allergic asthma. Sometimes the best choice for allergic asthma is simply inhaling peppermint oil. Frankincense deepens the breathing, while clary sage stops spastic coughing. Peppermint opens up the bronchials and sinuses, while chamomile and lavender relax them. Eucalyptus is generally contraindicated in cases of allergic asthma, but it is sometimes helpful in cases of nervous asthma. A good massage of the upper chest and back will encourage lymphatic drainage and help move chest congestion. Regular use of a chest and back massage should keep attacks at a minimum.

Asthma Rub for Children
2 drops frankincense
2 drops lavender
1 drop geranium
2 drop peppermint

Mix in 30 ml (2 tablespoons) of massage oil. Massage chest and back daily with blend.

Antispasmodic Asthma Rub
2 drops frankincense
1 drop Roman chamomile
2 drops clary sage
1 drop myrrh
optional: 1 drop peppermint

Mix in 2 teaspoons carrier oil and massage into upper chest and back.

Also try 2 drops each frankincense, clary sage and peppermint in a steam inhalation.

CONDITION: Bronchitis
ESSENTIAL OILS: Thyme linalol, frankincense, eucalyptus, peppermint, marjoram, myrrh, lavender, rosemary, tea tree, sandalwood, lemon
HERBS AND SUPPLEMENTS: IN-X, garlic, vitamin C, ALJ, mullein, ayurvedic bronchial formula, lobelia, four, pleurisy root, yerba santa

Bronchitis Inhalation
2 drops peppermint
3 drops eucalyptus
4 drops thyme linalol
2 drops clary sage or helichrysum
2 drops lavender

Use blend in nebulizing diffuser.

Brochitis Rub
8 drops frankincense
6 drops lemon
5 drops eucalyptus
3 drops oregano
1 ounce carrier oil

Massage on chest, bottom of feet and under toes. Place a hot compress on chest.

CONDITION: Coughs
ESSENTIAL OILS: Clary sage, eucalyptus, marjoram, myrrh, pine, rosemary, sandalwood
HERBS AND SUPPLEMENTS: Four, mullein, ALJ, garlic, herbs for colds and flu, LH

Vapor Balm for Coughs and Congestion
4 drops peppermint
8 drops eucalyptus
3 drops oregano
3 drops rosemary
1/2 ounce aloe vera gel
1/8 teaspoon massage oil

Combine ingredients and rub onto chest. Cover with a thin cotton cloth. Also try putting 3 drops of Tei Fu oil in 1 teaspoon of aloe gel and rubbing that onto the chest.

CONDITION: Sinusitis
ESSENTIAL OILS: Eucalyptus, tea tree, lavender, lemon, peppermint, pine, oregano
HERBS AND SUPPLEMENTS: Garlic, fenugreek, thyme, capsicum

Balm for the Sinuses
1 teaspoon golden salve
6 drops eucalyptus
3 drops peppermint
2 drops thyme

Blend together and apply a small amount to the inner nose daily.

The Urinary System

<u>KEY OILS:</u> **Roman chamomile, bergamot, sandalwood, tea tree, frankincense, lavender**

Although physicians in France use essential oils orally to treat urinary tract infections, this is not an option for the home user. Essential oils for this system are best used in aiding the elimination of excess fluids by stimulating the circulatory and lymphatic systems, and in cases of cystitis and inflammation.

**THERAPEUTIC ACTIONS OF OILS
FOR THE URINARY SYSTEM**

Anti-inflammatory—Reduces inflammation, irritation, and pain. **Oils:** Roman chamomile, lavender, sandalwood

Analgesic—Relieves pain and inflammation. **Oils:** Roman chamomile, peppermint, lavender, marjoram

Antimicrobial—Reduces the growth of unwanted microorganisms such as bacteria or yeast. **Oils:** Frankincense, lemon, bergamot, thyme linalol

---

Conditions and Therapeutic Treatments

CONDITION: Bladder Infection/Cystitis

HERBS AND SUPPLEMENTS: Corn silk, uva ursi, cranberry, buchu, marshmallow, horsetail, parsley, IN-X.

Soothing Cystitis Prevention Back Rub
5 drops bergamot
2 drops sandalwood
3 drops tea tree
3 drops lavender
1/2 ounce massage oil

Combine ingredients and rub into lower back. If you suspect an infection, add 2 drops thyme linalol or 1 drop frankincense.

Sitz baths with essential oils are often helpful. Use gentle oils such as bergamot, sandalwood, tea tree and thyme linalol (do not use any other type of thyme). Usually the E. coli bacteria is responsible for this uncomfortable condition. The best essential oils for fighting E. coli include cinnamon, bay laurel and clove. These are skin irritants and must be used with caution. They are not recommended in a sitz bath.

Sitz bath
2 drops tea tree
2 drops sandalwood
1 drop thyme linalol
2 drops lavender
1 teaspoon castile soap
2 Tablespoons apple cider vinegar

Mix the essential oils with the castile soap first; then add the soap mixture and the vinegar to your bath water. A sitz bath is one of the most appropriate methods for treating this condition, as it gets the remedy directly to the area needing healing. Fill a regular tub to hip level and sit in your "sitz" bath for 15 minutes.

CONDITION: Edema
3 drops geranium
4 drops pink grapefruit
4 drops rosemary
1 tablespoon aloe vera gel

Combine ingredients and rub into legs. These essential oils may also be combined in 1 tablespoon of honey and added to a running bath.

The Immune System

<u>KEY OILS:</u> **Thyme, oregano, tea tree, clove, lemon, rosemary**

Essential oils are part of a plant's immune system; that is, they provide protection against fungal blights, viral attacks and even parasites. Essential oils from plants are also effective against human pathogens. In fact, some oils have been found to be effective against antibiotic-resistant strains of bacteria. Essential oils are always appropriate in building and strengthening the immune system. Remember that antimicrobial properties are more concentrated in essential oils than in medicinal plants.

THERAPEUTIC ACTIONS OF ESSENTIAL OILS ON THE IMMUNE SYSTEM	
Antibiotics—Fights bacterial infection. **Oils:** Lemon, lavender, oregano, tea tree, thyme, bergamot, rosemary **Antivirals**—Fights viruses. **Oils:** Thyme, eucalyptus, marjoram, tea tree **Cytophylactics**—Increases white blood cell activity. **Oils:** Lemon, frankincense, lavender, rosemary, patchouli	**Antifungals**—Combats fungal infection. **Oils:** Tea tree, geranium, lavender, myrrh **Vulneraries**—Aids in the healing of wounds. **Oils:** Lavender, tea tree, marjoram, rosemary

Conditions and Therapeutic Treatments

CONDITION: Candida—See also recipes for yeast infection in glandular system and intestinal candida in the intestinal system.

ESSENTIAL OILS: Tea tree, eucalyptus, patchouli, peppermint, thyme, lavender, oregano.

HERBS AND SUPPLEMENTS: Acidophilus, bifidus, caprylic acid, grapefruit seed extract, garlic, pau d' arco, ginger, essential fatty acids, B-complex, Caprylimune, vitamin C, noni juice, olive leaf, olive oil.

Candida Immune-Booster Massage
2 ounces carrier oil
4 drops lemon
7 drops tea tree
5 drops thyme
3 drops rosemary
2 drops geranium
2 drops lavender

Combine ingredients in a glass container. Roll bottle between your hands to blend. Massage into skin daily.

CONDITION: Colds
ESSENTIAL OILS: Thyme, eucalyptus, cinnamon, clove, lavender, peppermint, pine, tea tree
HERBS AND SUPPLEMENTS: Garlic, echinacea, golden seal, olive leaf, vitamin C, colloidal silver, IN-X, CC-A, Nature's Immune Stimulator

Colds I
3 drops rosemary
2 drops peppermint
2 drops eucalyptus
3 drops lemon

Combine essential oils in an amber glass bottle. Use 3 to 4 drops in a steam inhalation.

Colds II
2 drops pine
2 drops clove
4 drops thyme
4 drops lemon
2 drops frankincense

Place essential oils in a nebulizing diffuser. Turn on the diffuser and sit close to it. Close your eyes and inhale deeply for about one minute. Do not allow diffuser to get close to the eyes. Never diffuse clove, oregano or cinnamon bark without closing your eyes, and never inhale for more than one or two minutes.

CONDITION: Cold Sores
ESSENTIAL OILS: Geranium, tea tree, thyme linalol, patchouli
HERBS AND SUPPLEMENTS: L-lysine, VS-C

Cold Sore Healer and Pain Relief
5 drops patchouli
10 drops geranium
15 drop sweet thyme (linalol only)

Mix essential oils together in a glass bottle. Add an equivalent amount of carrier oil. Apply directly to the cold sore with a Q-tip. You can add 2 drops of peppermint for additional pain relief.

Undiluted application of geranium on an emerging cold sore can also prevent it from breaking the surface and help it to heal in a few days' time.

CONDITION: Flu
ESSENTIAL OILS: Thyme linalol, eucalyptus, marjoram, tea tree
HERBS AND SUPPLEMENTS: Elderberry, colloidal silver, echinacea, golden seal, l-lysine, garlic

Flu Goo
4 drops thyme linalol
4 drops marjoram
3 drops eucalyptus
2 drops tea tree
2 drops oregano
1 teaspoon aloe vera gel
1/8 teaspoon massage oil

Combine ingredients and rub into chest before bed.

Fever-Reducing Compress
2 drops bergamot
1 drop lavender
1 drop eucalyptus

Add to 3 cups cool water. Swirl water to mix, then dip washcloth in water and apply this as a cool compress to the forehead.

The Glandular System

KEY OILS: **Geranium, clary sage, frankincense, rose, jasmine**

Essential oils can greatly support the glandular system, particularly the female reproductive system. They work on the glandular system largely through the sense of smell, which affects the hypothalamus and the pituitary gland, which, in turn, affect the hormones. Because this happens so quickly, using an essential oils spritzer can almost instantly alleviate certain hormonal concerns, such as hot flashes.

THERAPEUTIC ACTIONS OF ESSENTIAL OILS ON THE GLANDULAR SYSTEM	
Antispasmodics—Reduce muscular spasms and pain. Useful for painful periods and during labor. **Oils:** Roman chamomile, lavender, clary sage, marjoram **Aphrodisiacs**—Stimulate sexual interest. **Oils:** Jasmine, ylang ylang, rose, patchouli, sandalwood	**Emmenagogues**—Induce menstruation. Useful for loss of periods, normalizing menstruation and peri-menopause. **Oils:** Clary sage, rosemary **Hormonal**—Influence hormone levels. **Oils:** Clary sage, geranium, rose, frankincense

Conditions and Therapeutic Treatments

CONDITION: Aphrodisiacs

Jasmine, rose, ylang ylang, geranium, patchouli and sandalwood all act as aphrodisiacs. Their effectiveness depends to a great extent on wether the user enjoys the scent of the oil. All of the essential oils listed here blend well with each other. Use them to make a massage oil, to prepare a luxurious bath, or diffuse them in a tea light diffuser.

Sensual Honey Bath
2 drops jasmine
3 drops geranium
2 drops ylang ylang
3 drops sandalwood
2 drops clove
4 drops bergamot
1/4 cup runny honey

Mix the essential oils with the honey. Add honey mixture to a warm running bath.

CONDITION: Adrenal Support
ESSENTIAL OILS: Pine, spruce, lavender
HERBS AND SUPPLEMENTS: Vitamin C, B-complex, licorice

Be sure to check the thyroid, and add kelp or another iodine source to support the thyroid if necessary.

Adrenal Remedy
4 drops pine
2 drops lavender
1 drop Roman chamomile

Combine and rub into adrenal reflex points.

CONDITION: Cracked Nipples
HERBS AND SUPPLEMENTS: Essential fatty acids, B-complex, vitamin C

Cracked Nipples
4 drops rose
2 drops Roman chamomile
1 drops patchouli
2 teaspoons golden salve or 2 teaspoons extra virgin olive oil

Combine essential oils and salve or oil. Apply daily and cover area with a bandage.

CONDITION: Hot Flashes
ESSENTIAL OILS: Geranium, lavender, clary sage, pine
HERBS AND SUPPLEMENTS: Dong quai, Black cohosh, soy phytoestrogens, progesterone, wild yam, chaste tree, sage, red raspberry, vitamin E

Hot Flashes Spray
4 drops clary sage
3 drops Roman chamomile
3 drops geranium
1 drop pine
2 drops peppermint
2 drops lemon
4 ounces distilled water

Combine oils and water in a glass spritzer bottle. Shake to blend. Spritz and inhale to prevent or minimize hot flashes. Shake well before each use.

CONDITION: Impotence
ESSENTIAL OILS: Sandalwood, jasmine
HERBS AND SUPPLEMENTS: Yohimbe, zinc, B-complex

Remedy
Apply one drop of sandalwood to the area in question.

CONDITION: Leucorrhoea

Sitz bath
2 drops rosemary
3 drops thyme linalol
5 drops lavender
1 tablespoon Epsom salts or honey

Mix essential oils with Epsom salts or honey. Add to bath and soak for at least 15 minutes. Also try a douche with lavender and distilled water.

Lavender Douche
2 drops lavender
1 teaspoon apple cider vinegar
6 ounces purified water

Combine, shake, and use as douche.

CONDITION: Mastitis
Only the most gentle essential oils can be used for this condition.

Mastitis Rub
8 drops lavender
7 drops tea tree
5 drops Roman Chamomile
7 drops thyme linalol
10 drops mandarin
2 ounces massage oil

Combine ingredients and massage into both breasts and under the armpits three times daily. Apply one or two drops of lavender neat over the abscess area.

CONDITION: Painful Period
Useful oils include frankincense, marjoram, clary sage, Roman chamomile, geranium and neroli.

Painful Period Rub
2 drops chamomile
2 drops frankincense
1 drop clary sage
1 drop geranium
2 teaspoons aloe vera gel or massage oil

Mix essential oils with aloe or massage oil and massage into abdomen.

Painful Period with Heavy Flow
Use this blend several days before your period begins.

5 drops rose
5 drops frankincense
2 drops chamomile

Add essential oils to 1 ounce carrier oil, aloe vera gel or low-dose progesterone cream. Massage daily into abdomen and back.

CONDITION: PMS
ESSENTIAL OILS: Geranium, neroli, Roman chamomile, marjoram
HERBS AND SUPPLEMENTS: Pregesterone cream, dong quai, magnesium

PMS Aromatic Mood Adjuster
2 drops neroli
3 drops grapefruit
1 drop rose
2 drops sandalwood
1 teaspoon witch hazel
2 ounces distilled water

Combine in glass spritzer bottle. Shake before using.

CONDITION: Vaginitis and Yeast Infection
ESSENTIAL OILS: Lavender, tea tree, geranium, Roman chamomile

Vaginitis and Yeast Infection Salve
3 drops geranium
3 drops tea tree
3 drops lavender
2 drops chamomile
1 oz Golden Salve

Blend and apply a small amount with clean finger internally and externally. This will fight the infection and stop the itching. If skin is not sensitive, the essential oil concentration in this recipe can be doubled.

Yeast Infection
Place one drop each of lavender and tea tree on a natural tampon and insert. Leave in for 20 minutes.

Yeast Infection Douche
1 drop lavender
1 tablespoon plain, active, organic yogurt
1 quart of warm distilled water

Combine ingredients and use as a douche.

The Nervous System

<u>KEY OILS:</u> **Bergamot, chamomile, lavender, pink grapefruit, marjoram, neroli, rose**

Perhaps the most profound of all the effects of essential oils are manifest on the nervous system. No matter what condition you face, the mind–body connection should be addressed. Essential oils have the marvelous ability to shift the state of mind to a more peaceful and elevated state. And this shift happens in a matter of moments, whereas other methods—talking, therapy, etc.— usually take longer. Essential oils provide the mind with an instant release valve.

The process of understanding which oils affect emotions and how is a complicated one. Note which aromas appeal to you, then you can begin to heal your mind, emotions and body with aromatherapy.

THERAPEUTIC ACTIONS OF ESSENTIAL OILS ON THE NERVOUS SYSTEM

Anti-depressant—Uplifts the mind and moods. **Oils:** All citrus, geranium, rose
Euphoric—Causes a heightened state of excitement, happiness, or sensitivity, sometimes accompanied by a decrease sense of reality. **Oils:** Clary sage, rose
Hypnotic—Induces sleep. **Oils:** Neroli, chamomile, lavender
Nervine—Strengthens the nervous system. **Oils:** Lavender, patchouli, clary sage

Sedative—Calms an overcharged nervous system. **Oils:** Lavender, chamomile, marjoram, sandalwood, neroli
Stimulant—Brings energy or reaction to the nervous system; useful in combating fatigue and boredom. **Oils:** Lemon, peppermint, grapefruit, rosemary, eucaluptus
Tonic—Tones or balances to the entire system. **Oils:** Neroli, lavender

---

Conditions and Therapeutic Treatments

CONDITION: ADD/ADHD/Hyperactivity
ESSENTIAL OILS: Lavender, basil (Focus blend), lemon, pink grapefruit, Roman chamomile
HERBS AND SUPPLEMENTS: Calcium-magnesium, GABA, B-complex, pantothenic acid, l-cysteine, slippery elm or other bulk laxative.

Mix 10 drops lavender in 4 to 6 ounces of water in a spray bottle and spritz around the room. Shake before spritzing. Have the client smell various oils to determine which are soothing to him. Some children will prefer relaxing oils, while some will prefer stimulating oils.

Room Calming Mister
8 drops lavender
2 ounces purified water

Combine lavender and water in a glass spritzer bottle. Shake well and spritz around the room. Some teachers use this in the classroom while the children are at recess. Also try adding 6 drops of bergamot or 4 drops of mandarin to the lavender.

Hyperactivity Blend
8 drops lavender
4 drops chamomile
3 drops sandalwood
1 drop ylang ylang

Use in tea light diffuser. If you want to use this blend as a spritzer, mix the essential oils with 1/2 teaspoon witch hazel or vodka first, then add to 2 ounces of purified water in a misting spray bottle.

CONDITION: Alzheimer's

Diffusing rosemary can increase cerebral circulation. Use any aromas that may bring back memories, such as lemon, lavender and rosemary.

CONDITION: Anxiety
ESSENTIAL OILS: Bergamot, chamomile, clary sage, frankincense, lavender, neroli, rose, ylang ylang
HERBS AND SUPPLEMENTS: Calcium, magnesium, kava kava, B-complex, valerian, hops, chamomile, passionflower

Diffuse bergamot, lemon, lavender, ylang ylang or frankincense. Try sandalwood and chamomile together in a tea light diffuser. Clove can also be helpful, inhaled straight from the bottle. See recipes for stress.

CONDITION: Depression
ESSENTIAL OILS: : All citrus, peppermint, thyme, geranium, lavender. Almost any oil that personally appeals to you will be helpful.

Try diffusing any one of the following oils: Bergamot, lemon, grapefruit, lavender, geranium, ylang ylang, rose, peppermint, thyme.

Uplifting Roll-on
8 drops pink grapefruit
3 drops lemon
5 drops bergamot
1 drop neroli

Combine essential oils in a 10 ml roll-on bottle. Use on pulse points and remember to bring your wrist up to your nose throughout the day.

CONDITION: Headache and Migraine
ESSENTIAL OILS: Peppermint, lavender, pink grapefruit.
Lightly massage diluted essential oils into the temples and the hairline. Be sure not to get them close to the eyes, as this could aggravate the discomfort. For migraine headaches, lightly apply a small amount of peppermint oil in alcohol (I recommend vodka) to the forehead and temples. This may be too strong for some people. Check for neck and back tension as a possible cause.

Headache Oil
1 ounce massage oil
12 drops lavender
6 drops peppermint
4 drops eucalyptus

Mix the ingredients together. Use only a small amount on the temples, back of the head and top of the face just inside the hairline.

Neck and Shoulder Relief
10 drops lavender
7 drops marjoram
5 drops Roman chamomile
1 drop helichrysum

Mix the ingredients together. Use only a small amount on the temples, back of the head and top of the face just inside the hairline.

CONDITION: Insomnia
ESSENTIAL OILS: Lavender, marjoram, Roman chamomile, mandarin, neroli, rose, sandalwood
HERBS AND SUPPLEMENTS: Hops, valerian, skullcap, calcium–magnesium

Off to Sleep
3 drops neroli
6 drops lavender
4 drops marjoram
2 drops chamomile
3 drops bergamot

Combine essential oils in a nebulizing diffuser and diffuse overnight. Or add to the bath when combined with 1/4 cup Epsom salts or vegetable oil.

CONDITION: Jet Lag
ESSENTIAL OILS: Roman chamomile, clary sage, lavender, geranium, peppermint, marjoram
HERBS AND SUPPLEMENTS: Melatonin, passionflower, valerian

Jet Lag Bath
4 drops lavender
2 drops geranium
2 drops lemon

Mix with 1 teaspoon castile soap or Sunshine Concentrate. Add to running bath.

CONDITION: Meditation Aids
ESSENTIAL OILS: All woods and resins, frankincense, myrrh, sandalwood, rose

Mediation Blend I		*Meditation Blend II*
1 drop frankincense		2 drops frankincense
2 drops sandalwood	or	1 drop rose
		1 drop myrrh

Use either blend in tea light diffuser or aromaball. These blends are too thick for the nebulizing diffuser.

CONDITION: Mental Fatigue and Memory Loss
ESSENTIAL OILS: Clove, grapefruit, lemon, peppermint, pine, rosemary. Rosemary increases circulation to the brain, and lemon has been shown to increase concentration.
HERBS AND SUPPLEMENTS: Ginkgo, lecithin, Brain-Protex, selenium, B-Complex, free amino acids

Memory Aid
6 drops lemon
3 drops pink grapefruit
4 drops rosemary
2 drops peppermint

Combine ingredients. Put one or two drops on a tissue and inhale to enhance concentration. Or put several drops in an aromaball diffuser or a nebulizing diffuser.

Study Buddy
9 drops pink grapefruit
4 drops pine
2 drops rosemary

Combine oils. Put one or two drops on a tissue and inhale periodically. Or put several drops in an aromaball diffuser or a nebulizing diffuser.

CONDITION: Neuralgia, Neuropathy
ESSENTIAL OILS: Peppermint, helichrysum, geranium, clove, chamomile, lavender.
HERBS AND SUPPLEMENTS: B-vitamins, calcium, magnesium, MSM, potassium, progesterone cream, multivitamin, digestive enzymes, hops, valerian.

Neuralgia Oil
4 drops helichrysum
3 drops chamomile
3 drops lavender
2 drops geranium

Mix oils in 1 ounce of carrier oil and use for massage. If the neuralgia is not facial, add two drops of clove to the mixture. Try massaging the reflex points of the feet.

CONDITION: Stress
ESSENTIAL OILS: All citrus, especially bergamot, chamomile, lavender, clary sage, frankincense, geranium, marjoram, patchouli, rose, sandalwood, ylang ylang
HERBS AND SUPPLEMENTS: B-complex, vitamin C, free amino acids, passionflower, hops, dong quai, skullcap, valerian, chamomile, licorice

Stress Blend #1
5 drops bergamot
4 drops frankincense
3 drops grapefruit
2 drops neroli
2 drops clary sage

Count drops into a nebulizing diffuser, or dilute in 30 ml of oil for a wonderful massage.

Stress Blend #2
4 drops sandalwood
2 drops marjoram
2 drops thyme linalol
2 drops rose
1 drop geranium

Fill the basin of a tea light diffuser with water, and count drops of essential oil on top of the water. Light the tea light and enjoy.

The Muscular and Skeletal System

KEY OILS: **Helichrysum, marjoram, Roman chamomile, lavender, rosemary, eucalyptus, thyme linalol.**

Essential oils are useful in aiding the pain of arthritis and rheumatism. The also help with
inflammation of the joints and swelling of strained muscles, and improve local circulation.

THERAPEUTIC ACTIONS OF ESSENTIAL OILS ON THE MUSCULAR AND SKELETAL SYSTEM	
Anti-inflammatory—Reduce inflammation, irritation, pain, tenderness, and swelling. **Oils:** Roman chamomile, helichrysum, lavender, myrrh, geranium (for swelling). **Anti-toxic**—Help to detoxify the system of acid waste. **Oils:** Lemon, grapefruit, Cellutone	**Rubefacient**—Stimulate local circulation and thereby improve swelling, congestion, and inflammation. **Oils:** Deep Relief, rosemary, oregano

Conditions and Therapeutic Treatments

CONDITION: **Arthritis/Rheumatism**
ESSENTIAL OILS: Chamomile, eucalyptus, lavender, lemon, marjoram, oregano,
rosemary, thyme linalol

Arthritis Pain Relief
2 drops oregano
2 drops rosemary
1/2 teaspoon MSM/Glucosamine cream

*Squeeze cream into the palm of your hand. Add essential oils and rub into
painful joints.*

Icy Hot
4 drops deep relief blend
2 drops Tei Fu
1/8 teaspoon witch hazel
1 teaspoon healing AC cream

Combine ingredients and apply to affected areas.

CONDITION: Bursitis
ESSENTIAL OILS: Roman chamomile, lavender, peppermint

Bursitis Cream
10 drops lavender
2 drops peppermint
2 drops helichrysum
1 drop myrrh
1 ounce Healing AC cream

Mix ingredients and apply to affected areas.

CONDITION: Muscle Pain
ESSENTIAL OILS: Marjoram, lavender, Roman chamomile, helichrysum, eucalyptus, roremary
HERBS AND SUPPLEMENTS: Magnesium, calcium, amino acids, malic acid

Muscle Pain Bath
3 drops clary sage
2 drops Roman chamomile
1 drop helichrysum
5 drops lavender
2 cups Epsom salts (do not use with low blood pressure)

Combine the essential oils with the Epsom salts and add to a running bath.

Daytime After-Exercise Muscle Relief Rub
5 drops marjoram
4 drops rosemary
3 drops eucalyptus
2 drops peppermint
1 drop thyme

Add oils to 1/2 ounce carrier oil or aloe vera gel and rub into muscles.

Nighttime Muscle Relief Cream
5 drops marjoram
4 drops lavender
2 drop Roman chamomile
2 drops ylang ylang

Combine ingredients in 1/2 ounce of a cream base lotion, such as self-heal cream or Healing AC cream.

CONDITION: Rheumatism
ESSENTIAL OILS: Eucalyptus, helichrysum, rosemary, oregano, Roman chamomile

Rheumatism
2 drops rosemary
2 drops eucalyptus
1 drop helichrysum
3 drops lavender
1/4 teaspoon vodka
1/2 ounce Healing AC cream

Combine ingredients and apply to affected areas.

The Skin, Hair and Nails

<u>KEY OILS:</u> **Frankincense, helichrysum, lavender, patchouli, rosemary, rose, tea tree**

The use of essential oils can improve many concerns of the skin, hair and nails. For example, the antimicrobial properties of essential oils are helpful with lice. The increase in local circulation stimulated by essential oils exerts a helpful effect for hair loss. Many essential oils soothe the skin and help with rashes, eczema or other irritations.

Applying essential oils to the skin is one of the best ways to get them into the bloodstream. Diluting oils in a carrier oil improves and accelerates absorption into the body. Regular full-body massage helps reduce stress and increase circulation.

THERAPEUTIC ACTIONS OF ESSENTIAL OILS ON THE HAIR, SKIN AND NAILS

Anti-inflammatory—Reduces inflammation. **Oils:** Lavender, helichrysum, frankincense, geranium

Antimicrobial—Kills the small organisms that cause infections. All essential oils do this to some degree. **Oils:** Oregano, thyme, tea tree, lemon, eucalyptus

Cicatrizant—Accelerates the growth of healthy skin and helps prevent the formation of scars. **Oils:** Lavender, chamomile, helichrysum

Deodorant—Helps with bodily odors. **Oils:** Bergamot, thyme linalol, clary sage

Fungicidal—Kills fungus. Good for fungal toenails, athlete's foot and ringworm. **Oils:** Patchouli, thyme linalol, cinnamon, oregano, eucalyptus, tea tree, helichrysum, lemon, myrrh

Insect repellant—Deters insects. **Oils:** Geranium, clove, cinnamon leaf, peppermint, patchouli, pine, rosemary, lavender, eucalyptus

Vulnerary—Heals wounds. **Oils:** Frankincense, lavender, myrrh, geranium, lavender, tea tree

---

Conditions and Therapeutic Treatments

CONDITION: Acne
ESSENTIAL OILS: Tea tree, lavender, geranium, bergamot, frankincense, myrhh
HERBS AND SUPPLEMENTS: Liver cleansers, blood cleaners, SKN-AV

Lavender and/or tea tree can be applied neat with a Q-tip on individual blemishes. Try this blend for larger areas of the skin.

Acne Soother

7 drops lavender
5 drops tea tree
3 drops geranium
2 teaspoons aloe vera gel
1/8 teaspoon hazelnut or other high quality carrier oil.

Mix all ingredients and apply to troubled areas.

CONDITION: Athlete's Foot
ESSENTIAL OILS: Tea tree, thyme linalol, lavender, patchouli

4 drops tea tree
2 drops lavender
1/2 cup Epsom salts

Add to footbath and use daily. Follow with athlete's foot powder.

Athlete's Foot Powder

1/2 cup arrowroot powder
6 drops thyme linalol
5 drops lavender
4 drops tea tree
2 drops peppermint

Combine ingredients. Apply to feet and shake into shoes and socks. For nighttime gel, mix the same amount of essential oils as in powder recipe in 2 tablespoons of aloe gel. Do not use the arrowroot powder in the gel. Rub on feet before bed. Yield: three applications.

CONDITION: Boils
ESSENTIAL OILS: Eucalyptus, Roman chamomile, lavender, lemon, myrrh, thyme linalol, tea tree
HERBS AND SUPPLEMENTS: Echinacea, golden seal, garlic, colloidal silver, liquid chlorophyll, Vitamin A, proteolytic enzymes

Boil Oil

10 drops thyme linalol
5 drops eucalyptus
5 drops myrrh
5 drops lavender
1 teaspoon colloidal silver
2 teaspoons Golden Salve
1 capsule garlic oil
1 capsule vitamin E

Mix ingredients and apply to the affected area several times a day. Be sure to wash your hands before and after application.

CONDITION: Bruises
ESSENTIAL OILS: Lavender, helichrysum, geranium
HERBS AND SUPPLEMENTS: Vitamin C with bioflavonoids, alfalfa, leafy green vegetables, co-enzyme Q-10

Bruise Healer

8 drops helichrysum
7 drops lavender
3 drops geranium

Mix oils in 1 teaspoon carrier oil or 1/2 ounce of healing cream with arnica. Apply several times a day. Diligent application of this blend will cause the bruise to heal much more quickly with less discoloration of the skin.

CONDITION: Bug Bites

Neat lavender or tea tree will stop the itching and help clear the irritation. The relief should last about three hours.

CONDITION: Burns

Apply lavender oil neat. See also sunburn.

CONDITION: Cellulite
ESSENTIAL OILS: Cellu-Tone blend
HERBS AND SUPPLEMENTS: Lecithin, kelp, bladderwrack, vitamin C

Cellulite Formula
3 drops grapefruit
2 drops geranium
2 drops lemon
2 drops thyme
1 drop oregano

Add oils to 1 tablespoon massage oil or aloe vera gel. Massage into cellulite once daily after showering and skin brushing. Increase your exercise levels. Try using the detoxification bath three times weekly.

CONDITION: Cold Sores
ESSENTIAL OILS: Patchouli, geranium, thyme linalol
HERBS AND SUPPLEMENTS: L-lysine, Vitamin C

Apply geranium neat to the area when the first tingle of a cold sore is felt. Applied several times a day, this may prevent the cold sore from erupting. Otherwise, this recipe helps kill the virus, numb the pain and aids the healing of the skin around the cold sore.

CONDITION: Cracked and Calloused Heels

Heel Healer
3 drops patchouli
1/2 teaspoon lotion base or healing cream with calendula

Combine the lotion and the patchouli. Apply liberally to heels. Cover with cotton socks overnight. Repeat as long as necessary. A drop of peppermint can be added to cool the feet, if desired.

CONDITION: **Cracked Nipples**

> 1 tablespoon (15 ml) extra virgin olive oil
> 4 drops rose
> 5 drops lavender
> 3 drops chamomile

Combine in a glass bottle and apply as needed. These oils can also be combined with 1 tablespoon of healing cream with calendula.

CONDITION: **Cuts**

> Apply lavender or tea tree neat.

CONDITION: **Deodorant**

Use 1–2 drops lavender neat under each arm. Or mix 2–3 drops geranium in aloe vera gel or pau d'arco lotion and apply under arms. For extremely stressful days, try 2 drops thyme linalol and 1 drop of lemon mixed in pau d'arco lotion.

> ***Deodorant Spray***
> 1/2 ounce apple cider vinegar
> 3 ounces R.O. or distilled water
> 1 teaspoon witch hazel
> 30 drops of essential oils of your choice. Or use mine: 7 drops thyme, 3 drops geranium, 5 drops lavender, 3 drops peppermint, 4 drops lemon, 3 drops sandalwood, 2 drops clove, 3 drops tea tree

Combine ingredients in a 4-ounce glass spray bottle. Use as needed.

CONDITION: **Dandruff**
ESSENTIAL OILS: Lavender, thyme linalol, eucalyptus, peppermint, rosemary
HERBS AND SUPPLEMENTS: Horsetail, kelp, B-complex, evening primrose oil or flax seed oil.

Vinegar Rinse
4 drops lavender
3 drops thyme linalol
2 drops eucalyptus or peppermint
2 drops rosemary
1 tablespoon apple cider vinegar
1 ounce distilled water

Mix oils with vinegar. Then combine with water. Massage about one teaspoon of mixture into the scalp before bed. The smell of the vinegar will dissipate in a few minutes. Also try rinsing the hair with nettle tea after washing.

CONDITION: **Eczema**

Eczema Cool Compress
1 drop bergamot
1 drop lemon
2 drops chamomile
2 drops lavender
6 ounces cool water
1 small cotton cloth (washed, unused cloth diapers will work)

Combine oils and water in a glass bowl and stir. Soak cloth in water, wring out and apply to skin. When cloth becomes warm, repeat the process. Continue for 15 minutes or until itching and irritation is reduced.

Eczema Healing Oil
3 capsules vitamin E (cut open)
3 capsules evening primrose oil (cut open)
1 drop rose oil
2 drops helichrysum
2 drops chamomile
2 drops geranium
1 drop myrrh
2 drops tea tree
1/4 teaspoon rose hip seed oil
1 tablespoon virgin organic olive oil or flax seed oil

Combine and apply three times daily.

CONDITION: Fungus
ESSENTIAL OILS: Tea tree, geranium, lemon, thyme linalol
HERBS AND SUPPLEMENTS: Pau d'arco, acidophilus, bifidus, grapefruit seed extract, Caprylic Acid, Multivitamin, Vitamin C, Enteric Coated Garlic.

Fungal Footbath See also recipe for toenail fungus.
1 drop tea tree
1 drop geranium
1 drop lemon
2 drops thyme linalol

Mix with 1/2 cup dead sea salts in warm footbath. Soak for 10 minutes.

CONDITION: Toenail Fungus

Apply tea tree and lavender alternately neat three times a day. If the toenail does not respond, try the following recipe:
9 drops thyme linalol
5 drops geranium
4 drops lemon
3 drops sandalwood
2 drops patchouli

Combine essential oils with an equal volume of massage oil or extra virgin olive oil. Apply to affected nail twice daily, and cover with bandage at night.

CONDITION: Hair Loss (premature)
ESSENTIAL OILS: Lavender, rosemary, thyme linalol, clary sage
HERBS AND SUPPLEMENTS: B-complex with extra B6, horsetail, alfalfa, silica, multivitamin, flax seed oil, evening primrose oil

Lavender has been shown to help reverse hair loss. Traditional remedies for hair loss include rosemary and sage. Don't forget to investigate the possibility of hair loss due to toxic load or hormone imbalance.

Scalp Treatment
1 drop lavender
1 drop clary sage or rosemary
1/8 teaspoon jojoba oil

Combine ingredients and massage into scalp before bedtime.

Thinning Hair Help
5 drops lavender
2 drops rosemary
3 drops thyme linalol
1 teaspoon jojoba oil

Combine the essential oils with the jojoba oil in a glass bottle. Hold the bottle in your hands and rub it back and forth to warm and blend the oils. Allow the oils to sit overnight on the scalp. After shampooing your hair in the morning, you may want to rinse your hair with 1 tablespoon apple cider vinegar diluted with 2 cups water.

Precautions: Some people have more sensitive skin than others. Test this recipe on a small area of the scalp before applying all over.

CONDITION: Lice

The best oils for the treatment of lice include tea tree, rosemary, oregano and thyme. Geranium, citronella and lemongrass may also provide help.

Lice Shampoo
15 ml of tea tree or thyme linalol (not both)
15-ounce bottle of shampoo

Mix oil with shampoo and use as normal. Be sure to keep shampoo out of the eyes.

Lice Scalp Treatment 1
14 drops tea tree
5 drops thyme linalol
1 teaspoon carrier oil
1 teaspoon jojoba oil

Rub mixture into the scalp. Place a shower cap over the hair and allow this blend to sit for several hours, according to skin sensitivity.

Lice Scalp Treatment 2
7 drops tea tree
7 drops thyme linalol
3 drops rosemary
5 drops geranium
2 drops oregano
1 teaspoon jojoba oil
2 teaspoons carrier oil

Blend the essential oils with the jojoba and carrier oils. Massage a small amount into the scalp before bed. Wear a shower cap over your hair and keep this treatment on the head in order to kill the eggs and nits.

CONDITION: Psoriasis
ESSENTIAL OILS: Roman chamomile, lavender, helichrysum, bergamot, geranium, clary sage
HERBS AND SUPPLEMENTS: Essential fatty acids, liver cleansers, reduce chemical bond

Baths in Dead Sea salts can provide great relief.

Soothing Bath
2 drops chamomile
4 drops clary sage
1 drop helichrysum
2 drops bergamot
2 cups dead sea salts

Combine oils and salts. Add to bath and soak for 30 minutes.

Soothing Skin Oil
1 ounce jojoba oil
1/2 ounce carrier, hazelnut or rice bran oil
3 capsules of vitamin E, cut open
3 drops sandalwood
3 drops bergamot
2 drops ylang ylang
2 drops myrrh
2 drops clary sage
1 drop tea tree
1 drop pine

Apply to affected areas as needed. Omit bergamot if you will be exposed to the sun.

CONDITION: Ringworm
ESSENTIAL OILS: Eucalyptus, grapefruit, lemon, patchouli, tea tree

Ringworm Treatment
2 drops patchouli
5 drops geranium
7 drops lavender
15 drops tea tree
2 capsules vitamin E
1 tablespoon vegetable oil or Golden Salve

Mix essential oils and vitamin E into vegetable oil. Apply with a Q-tip to the affected area three times daily. Also try the fungal footbath recipe.

CONDITION: Scarring
ESSENTIAL OILS: Helichrysum, lavender, frankincense, myrhh, rose, geranium

Scar massage oil
2 tablespoons flax seed oil
1 teaspoon jojoba oil
10 capsules vitamin E oil
5 drops geranium
4 drops rose
4 drops frankincense
3 drops myrrh
2 drops helichrysum

Apply blend to healing wound twice daily to prevent scarring.

CONDITION: Sunburn
ESSENTIAL OILS: Helichrysum, lavender, frankincense, myrhh, rose,

Sunburn Soother
4 ounces plain, organic yogurt, cold from the refrigerator
25 drops lavender
8 drops helichrysum
5 drops geranium
4 drops chamomile

Mix in a glass container with a wooden spoon. Apply to sunburned skin. Try adding 4 drops of eucalyptus to the blend. Keep refrigerated. This mixture will stay fresh for about a week.

Sunburn Spray
1.5 ounces purified water
1/2 teaspoon vodka
1 tablespoon aloe vera gel
50 drops lavender

Combine all ingredients in a 2-ounce glass spritzer bottle. Shake before each use. Keep it in the refrigerator for extra cooling effect.

After-Sun Treatments

Lavender essential oil may accelerate the rate at which the skin repairs itself, and it will lessen the pain and heat of sunburn. While some people recommend putting lavender directly on a sunburn I prefer to mix it with aloe vera first.

Cooling Lavender Spray with Aloe
2 teaspoons aloe vera gel
30 drops lavender essential oil
6 drops peppermint
1 teaspoon vodka
7 teaspoons reverse osmosis or distilled water
1 teaspoon massage oil (optional, if skin is tight)

Squeeze the aloe vera gel into a glass spritzer bottle. Next, add the lavender and peppermint essential oils and the vodka. Add the water and shake thoroughly. Mist the burn lightly with this spritzer.

CONDITION: Thread Veins
ESSENTIAL OILS: Rose, lavender

Thread Veins and Tender Skin
2 drops rose
3 drops lavender
4 teaspoon witch hazel
2 ounces rose water

Combine and apply to cheeks twice a day. Also use as a cool compress.

CONDITION: Wounds

Wound Healer
1 drop frankincense
2 drops geranium
2 drops lavender
1/4 teaspoon beeswax base ointment (golden salve)

Mix oils with ointment and apply to wound two to three times daily. Cover with a bandage between applications. If the wound is oozing and needs to be dried, place 1 drop of tea tree on the bandage, or drop it neat onto the wound if there is no skin sensitivity to tea tree.

10

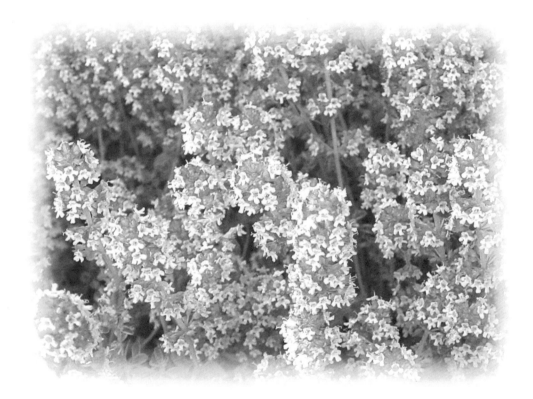

Additional Materials

GLOSSARY

Abortifacient: ....Capable of inducing abortions.

Amenorrhea: ....Abnormal absence of menstruation outside pregnancy in pre-menopausal women.

Analgesic: ....A pain-killing substance or remedy.

Anaphrodisiac: ....Inhibits or discourages sexual desire.

Antibiotic: ....Substances that inhibit or kill microorganisms.

Anthelmintic: ....An agent that destroys or expels worms.

Antiphlogisitic: ....A substance that reduces or fights inflammation.

Antipruritic: ....Relieves itching.

Antipuetretactive: ....Prevents the bacterial decomposition of tissue.

Antiseptic: ....Prevents or arrests the growth of microorganisms.

Antispasmodic: ....Capable of preventing or relieving spasms or convulsions.

Antitussive: ....Prevents or relieves coughs.

Aphrodisiac: ....A substance that arouses sexual desire.

Arrhythmia: ....An alteration in rhythm of the heartbeat.

Arteriosclerosis: ....A chronic disease characterized by abnormal thickening and hardening of the arterial walls with resulting loss of elasticity.

Arthritis: ....Acute or chronic inflammation of the joints due to infection or metabolic conditions.

Bactericide: ....A substance that destroys bacteria.

Bacteriostatic: ....Inhibition of the growth of bacteria without their destruction.

Bilious: ....Marked by or suffering from liver dysfunction and especially excessive secretion of bile.

Cardiotonic: ....Tones the heart muscle.

Carminative: ....An agent that causes the expelling of gas from the intestine so as to relieve colic or griping.

Catarrh: ....Inflammation of a mucous membrane.

Cholagogue: ....An agent that aids in the elimination of bile from the gall-bladder and bile ducts.

Cicatrizing: ....Scar formation at the site of a healing wound.

Colic: ....A paroxysm of acute abdominal pain localized in a hollow organ and often caused by spasm, obstruction, or twisting.

Colitis: ....Inflammation of the colon.

Congestion: ....An excessive fullness of the blood vessels in an organ.

Cystitis: ....Inflammation of the bladder.

Depurative: ....An agent that fights impurities in the blood or organs.

Diaphoretic: ....An agent that causes sweating or perspiration.

Digestive: ....A substance that helps stimulate digestion.

Diuretic: ....Tending to increase the flow of urine.

Dysmenorrhea: ....Painful menstruation.

Dyspepsia: ....Painful digestion.

Dyspepnea: ....Painful or difficult breathing.

Edema: ....An abnormal infiltration and excess accumulation of serous fluid in connective tissue or in a serous cavity.

Emetic: ....An agent that induces vomiting.

Emmenagogue: ....An agent that promotes menstrual discharge.

Emollient: ....A substance that soothes and softens tissues and reduces inflammation.

Emphysema: ....A condition of the lung marked by abnormal dilation of its air spaces and distension of its walls and frequently by impairment of heart action.

Eupeptic: ....A substance that aids digestion.

Febrifuge: ....An agent that reduces fever.

Flatulence: ....Characterized by excess gas in the stomach and intestine.

Galactagogue: ....An agent that promotes the production of milk.

Hepatic: ....Of, relating to, affecting, associated with, supplying, or draining the liver.

Hypertension: ....Abnormally high blood pressure, especially arterial blood pressure.

Hypertensive: ....An agent that raises blood pressure.

Hypnotic: ....A sleep-inducing agent.

Hypotensive: ....An agent that lowers blood pressure.

Leukocyte: ....A white blood cell.

Leukorrhea: ....A whitish discharge from the vagina resulting from inflammation or congestion of the mucous membrane.

Neuralgia: ....Acute, stabbing pain radiating along the course of one or more nerves.

Neuritis: ....Inflammation of a nerve.

Nervine: ....Supports the nervous system.

Pneumonia: ....A disease of the lungs characterized by inflammation.

Psoriasis: ....A chronic skin disease characterized by circumscribed red patches covered with white scales.

Purgative: ....An agent that produces evacuation or movement of the bowels.

Rubefacient: ....A substance for external application that produces redness of the skin.

Stomachic: ....A stimulant or tonic for the stomach.

Sudorific: ....An agent that causes sweating or perspiration.

Vasoconstrictor: ....An agent that induces constriction of the blood vessels.

Vasodilator: ....An agent that induces an enlargement or dilation of the blood vessels.

Vermifuge: ....An agent that destroys or expels worms.

Vulnerary: ....A substance that is useful in healing wounds.

References and Recommended Reading

Cooksley, Valerie Gennari. *Aromatherapy—A Lifetime Guide to Healing Essential Oils.* Prentice Hall, N.J., 1996. ISBN 0-13-349432-2.

Damian, Peter and Kate. *Aromatherapy Scent and Psyche.* Healing Arts Press, Rochester, Vt., 1995. ISBN 0-89281-530-2

Davis, Patricia. *Aromatherapy, an A-Z.* CW Daniel Company, United Kingdom, 1995. ISBN 0-85207-295-3

De Amicis, Ralph and Lahni. *Feng Shui and the Tango in Twelve Easy Lessons.* Cuore Libre Publishing, Bryn Athyn, Pa., 2001. orders@cuorelibrepublishing.com.

Edwards, Victoria. *The Aromatherapy Companion.* ISBN 1-5801-7150-8

Fischer-Rizzi, Susanne. *Complete Aromatherapy Handbook.* Sterling Publishing, New York, 1990. ISBN 0-8069-8222-5

Herb Allure. *HART Aromatherapy.* herballure.com

Howe, Maggy. "The Healing Rose." *Country Living Magazine,* June 2000, 86.

Jones, Larissa "Is Yous Home Safe?" Evergreen Aromatherapy, 2001.

Keville, Kathy and Green, Mindy. *Aromatherapy—A Complete Guide to the Healing Art.* The Crossing Press, Freedom, Calif., 1995. ISBN 0-89594-692-0

Lawless, Julie. *Aromatherapy and the Mind.* Thorsons, San Fransisco, 1994. ISBN 0-7225-2927-9

Lawless, Julie. *The Complete Illustrated Guide to Aromatherapy.* Barnes and Noble, New York, 1997. ISBN 0-7607-0703-0.

Lawless, Julie. *The Illustrated Encyclopedia of Essential Oils.* Barnes and Noble, New York, 1995. ISBN 1-852530-721-8.

Mojay, Gabriel. *Aromatherapy for Healing the Spirit*. Healing Arts Press, Rochester, VT., 1997. ISBN 0-89281-887-5.

Price, Shirley. *Aromatherapy Workbook*. Thorsons, San Fransisco, 1993. ISBN 0-7225-2645-8

Schnaubelt, Kurt. *Advanced Aromatherapy*. Healing Arts Press, Rochester, Vt., 1998. ISBN 0-89281-743-7

Tisserand, Robert. *Essential Oil Safety*. Churchill Livingstone, New York, 1995. ISBN 0-443-05260-3

Tucker, Arthur O. "The Therapy of Aroma." *Herbs for Health*, Jan/Feb 1999.

Valnet, Jean. *The Practice of Aromatherapy*. The Healing Arts Press, Rochester, VT., 1990. ISBN 0-89281-398-9

Walji, Hasnain, Ph.D. *The Healing Power of Aromatherapy*. Prima Publishing, Rocklin, Calif., 1996. ISBN 0-7615-0441-9

Watson, Franzeca. *Aromatherapy Blends and Remedies*. Thorsons, San Fransisco, 1995. ISBN 0-72255-3222-9

Wilson, Roberta. *Aromatherapy for Vibrant Health and Beauty*. Avery Publishing, New York, 1995. ISBN 0-89529-627-6.

Worwood, Valerie Ann. *The Complete Book of Essential Oils and Aromatherapy*. New World Library, Novato, Calif., 1991. ISBN 0-931432-82-0

Abbreviated Index

Larissa Jones

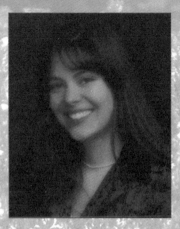

Larissa Jones is a master aromatherapist, herbalist, and public speaker. She has worked in the health industry for seven years, teaching seminars for the past five years across the United States, Canada, and Europe on herbal remedies, natural healing, and complementary medicine. In 1999 she completed a master's aromatherapy course taught by one of the most internationally respected people in the field, Dr. Kurt Schnaubelt. She completed 120 hours of coursework and case studies with renowned aromatherapist Victoria Edwards. In 1998 she continued her studies at the Third Annual International Scientific Aromatherapy Symposium in France.

In France, Larissa met with scientists and researchers from the French National Center for Biomedicine at the University of Perpignan, where she studied the latest research on detection of adulteration, quality control of essential oils, and the relationship between climate and essential oil characteristics.

As a Corporate Regional Manager for Nature's Sunshine Products in Provo, Utah, Larissa helped create and launch the company's first aromatherapy school. In addition, she worked closely with Steven Horne in creating the School of Natural Health, which teaches students to correlate symptoms with correct herbal supplements. The schools incorporate the latest research on herbs and essential oils, while making the art of aromatherapy accessible to all.

TO ORDER *additional copies of* Aromatherapy for Body, Mind, and Spirit, *please fill out this form and mail it to:*

Evergreen Aromatherapy
2096 East Evergreen Ave.
Salt Lake City, Utah 84109

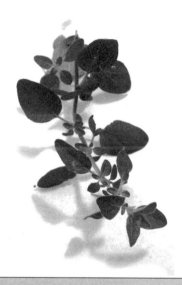

Quantity _____

Price each _____

Subtotal _____

Utah residents add 6.6% sales tax _____

Shipping and handling _____

TOTAL ENCLOSED _____

PRICING:

1–3 copies	$19.95 each U.S. ($27.20 Canadian)
4–10 copies	$17.95 each U.S. ($24.48 Canadian)
11+ copies	$15.00 each U.S. ($26.25 Canadian)

SHIPPING:

1– 3 copies	$3.00
4–10 copies	$6.50
11+ copies	$12.00

Name _____

Mailing/Shipping Address_____

Phone_____   email _____

Please make check payable to Evergreen Aromatherapy.
Please allow 4 to 8 weeks for delivery.